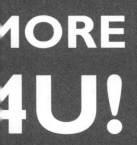

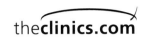
theclinics.com

# ORAL AND MAXILLOFACIAL SURGERY CLINICS
## of North America

The Role of the Oral and Maxillofacial Surgeon in Wartime, Emergencies, and Terrorist Attacks

DAVID B. POWERS, DMD, MD
Guest Editor

RICHARD H. HAUG, DDS
Consulting Editor

August 2005  •  Volume 17  •  Number 3

**SAUNDERS**

An Imprint of Elsevier, Inc.
PHILADELPHIA    LONDON    TORONTO    MONTREAL    SYDNEY    TOKYO

**W.B. SAUNDERS COMPANY**
*A Division of Elsevier Inc.*

1600 John F. Kennedy Blvd., Suite 1800, Philadelphia, PA 19103-2899

http://www.oralmaxsurgery.theclinics.com

**ORAL AND MAXILLOFACIAL SURGERY**
**CLINICS OF NORTH AMERICA**                                  Volume 17, Number 3
**August 2005**                                                  ISSN 1042-3699
Editor: John Vassallo                                        ISBN 1-4160-2840-4

*Oral and Maxillofacial Surgery Clinics of North America* (ISSN 1042-3699) is published quarterly by W.B. Saunders Company. Corporate and editorial offices: Elsevier, Inc., 1600 John F. Kennedy Blvd., Suite 1800, Philadelphia, PA 19103-2899. Accounting and circulation offices: 6277 Sea Harbor Drive, Orlando, FL 32887-4800. Periodicals postage paid at Orlando, FL 32862, and additional mailing offices. Subscription prices are $180.00 per year for US individuals, $280.00 per year for US institutions, $90.00 per year for US students and residents, $208.00 per year for Canadian individuals, $325.00 per year for Canadian institutions, $225.00 per year for international individuals, $325.00 per year for international institutions and $113.00 per year for Canadian and foreign students/residents. To receive student/resident rate, orders must be accompanied by name or affiliated institution, date of term, and the *signature* of program/residency coordinator on institution letterhead. Orders will be billed at individual rate until proof of status is received. Foreign air speed delivery is included in all *Clinics* subscription prices. All prices are subject to change without notice. POSTMASTER: Send address changes to *Oral and Maxillofacial Surgery Clinics of North America,* W.B. Saunders Company, Periodicals Fulfillment, Orlando, FL 32887-4800. **Customer Service: 1-800-654-2452 (US). From outside of the US, call 1-407-345-4000.**

Printed in the United States of America.

# CONSULTING EDITOR

**RICHARD H. HAUG, DDS,** Professor of Oral and Maxillofacial Surgery; and Executive Associate Dean, University of Kentucky College of Dentistry, Lexington, Kentucky

# GUEST EDITOR

**DAVID B. POWERS, DMD, MD,** Program Director, Oral and Maxillofacial Surgery Residency, Wilford Hall Medical Center, Lackland Air Force Base, Texas

# CONTRIBUTORS

**SHAN K. BAGBY, DMD,** Assistant Director, Oral and Maxillofacial Surgery Residency, Brooke Army Medical Center, Fort Sam Houston, Texas

**SIDNEY L. BOURGEOIS, Jr, DDS,** Staff, Department of Oral and Maxillofacial Surgery; and Faculty, National Capital Consortium, National Naval Medical Center, Bethesda, Maryland

**MICHAEL J. DOHERTY, DDS,** Chief Resident, Department of Oral and Maxillofacial Surgery, National Capital Consortium, National Naval Medical Center, Bethesda, Maryland

**COLLEEN M. FITZPATRICK, MD,** Resident, Department of General Surgery, Wilford Hall Medical Center, Lackland Air Force Base, Texas

**TAMER GOKSEL, DDS, MD,** Assistant Program Director, Oral and Maxillofacial Surgery Service, Brooke Army Medical Center, Fort Sam Houston, Texas

**OSCAR HASSON, DDS,** Senior Surgeon, Department of Oral and Maxillofacial Surgery, Kaplan Medical Center, Rehovot, Israel

**HOLLY D. HATT, DMD, MD,** Program Director, Oral and Maxillofacial Surgery Residency, National Naval Medical Center, San Diego, California

**JEFFREY D. KERBY, MD, PhD,** Associate Professor, Department of Surgery, University of Alabama at Birmingham, Birmingham, Alabama

**BRENT KINCAID, DDS,** Staff Oral and Maxillofacial Surgeon, United States Air Force Academy, Colorado Springs, Colorado

**ROBERT K. McGHEE, DDS,** Chief Resident, Department of Oral and Maxillofacial Surgery, Wilford Hall Medical Center, Lackland Air Force Base, Texas

**CHRISTOPHER C. MEDLEY, DDS, MD,** Consultant to the Air Force Surgeon General for Oral and Maxillofacial Surgery, Wilford Hall Medical Center, Lackland Air Force Base, Texas

**DAVID B. POWERS, DMD, MD,** Program Director, Oral and Maxillofacial Surgery Residency, Wilford Hall Medical Center, Lackland Air Force Base, Texas

**DARON C. PRAETZEL, DMD,** Chief Resident, Department of Oral and Maxillofacial Surgery, Wilford Hall Medical Center, Lackland Air Force Base, Texas

**O. BAILEY ROBERTSON, DDS,** Chief of Facial Plastic and Cosmetic Surgery, Oral and Maxillofacial Surgery Residency, Wilford Hall Medical Center, Lackland Air Force Base, Texas

**JOHN P. SCHMITZ, DDS, PhD,** San Pedro Facial Surgery; and Professor, Department of Orthopaedics, University of Texas Health Sciences Center, San Antonio, Texas

**CHARLES G. STONE, Jr, DDS,** Chief Resident, Department of Oral and Maxillofacial Surgery, National Capital Consortium, Walter Reed Army Medical Center, Washington, District of Columbia

**MICHAEL J. WILL, DDS, MD,** Chief, Oral and Maxillofacial Surgery; Consultant, United States Army Surgeon General; and Program Director, National Capital Consortium, Walter Reed Army Medical Center, Washington, District of Columbia

# CONTENTS

concept has been several decades in the making, and with products in phase III clinical trials, the use of hemoglobin-based oxygen carriers may be close to reality. The potential applications are limitless with interest from the military and civilian sectors.

Success in accurately diagnosing and providing first-contact treatment for patients with facial burns relies on accurate history taking, physical examination, and close observation. Providers must understand the early and delayed effects of heat on human tissue and the respiratory system. Initial treatment should be aimed at preventing complications and accurately identifying the extent of injury and rapidly administering appropriate therapy. Vigilance is important given the delayed nature of edema caused by burns. Rapid diagnosis and early intervention are key in keeping patients alive and facilitating definitive burn care.

Terrorist attacks have been occurring in Israel since the early 1970s. Israeli oral and maxillofacial surgeons are involved in the treatment of victims, because facial injuries are generally present after these attacks. Facial wounds are caused by blocks and stone throwing, stabbings, gunshots, and suicide bombings. The characteristics of each type of injury and their treatment are described.

Improvised explosive devices have created a new class of casualties that presents a unique surgical challenge for oral and maxillofacial surgeons. The injury pattern and severity are different from those seen in conventional trauma patients. Because of battlefield circumstances, patients are sometimes delayed significantly in their transport to a trauma center, and they frequently arrive at a trauma center with hypotension, hypothermia, and acidosis. Definitive care is delayed while the hemodynamic status and life-threatening injuries are stabilized. Hospital triage protocols must be well established in advance to prepare a timely response to the mass casualty event. Proper resource use is an ever-evolving challenge for hospital staff during these times.

The treatment of injuries from a nuclear weapon or a radioactive dispersal device most likely will be in a mass casualty scenario. Radiation injuries complicate the treatment process, with increased emphasis on early intervention. The care of patients must proceed in an orderly fashion. If radiation injury occurs as part of a mass casualty, some organized method of triage, decontamination, evacuation, and treatment must be implemented. Oral and maxillofacial surgeons should plan to become integral members of the treatment team, especially considering their wide scope of training. It is important for all health care providers to become familiar with the types of injuries that can be expected after a radiologic attack and the treatment modalities that can preserve life should such a catastrophe occur.

# FORTHCOMING ISSUES

# PREVIOUS ISSUES

---

## THE CLINICS ARE NOW AVAILABLE ONLINE!

Access your subscription at:
**www.theclinics.com**

---

ELSEVIER
SAUNDERS

Oral Maxillofacial Surg Clin N Am 17 (2005) ix – x

**ORAL AND
MAXILLOFACIAL
SURGERY CLINICS**
of North America

Foreword

# The Role of the Oral and Maxillofacial Surgeon in Wartime, Emergencies, and Terrorist Attacks

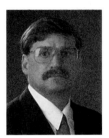

Richard H. Haug, DDS
*Consulting Editor*

It is ironic that during periods of armed conflict, there are not only devastation and destruction but also rapid advances and improvements in medicine and surgery. This observation seems to be consistent throughout the ages. The Napoleonic Wars contributed aggressive wound débridement (and amputation) to the surgical armamentarium. The Crimean War refined this concept of aggressive débridement, especially in the maxillofacial region, to preservation of tissues. The American Civil War brought camp and hospital sanitation into focus. World War I contributed early resuscitation and early treatment at base hospitals to the principals of casualty management. World War II provided a focus on the administrative preparation for managing wounded personnel. Blood transfusions, hydration, and antibiotic therapy were foci of World War II medical and surgical management that made a great impact on the survival of injured persons. The Korean War contributed external fixation and mobile hospital units. The Vietnam War contributed medical and surgical evacuation, especially via helicopters, to our improved understanding of the management and increased survival of injured patients. The improvements in biomedical and scientific

progress during armed conflicts have been observed to occur in the following three phases: (1) a latent period, (2) one of rapid and diverse advances, and (3) a period of consolidation of ideas and application of these developments into clinical practice.

Once again we find ourselves involved in another armed conflict in the Middle East. With this conflict are associated new concepts in warfare and new terms to describe these issues. Only conceptual solutions and phase two advances are currently available to us. In an attempt to provide "cutting edge" knowledge to the readers of the *Oral and Maxillofacial Surgery Clinics of North America*, this issue is devoted to a consolidation of observations and advances in the delivery of care resulting from the Iraqi conflict. The authors assembled for this issue possess the highest caliber of character and are among the brightest and most competent surgeons that our specialty has to offer. I can state this opinion through close personal observation, having had the honor to examine some of these surgeons on their "boards," having participated in lectures and seminars with many, having site visited their bases and training programs, and having observed the results of the surgical management provided by these outstanding in-

doi:10.1016/j.coms.2005.05.004

dividuals. Some of the topics covered in this issue are relatively new to our literature, such as bioterrorism and nuclear terrorism. Some articles relate improvements in medical and surgical management, such as care of the burned and management of victims of explosions. Finally, some articles are consolidations of observations and management techniques into algorithms or summary articles. I am certain that readers of this issue will be intrigued and challenged, and come away with state-of-the-art knowledge.

Richard H. Haug, DDS
*Department of Oral and Maxillofacial Surgery*
*University of Kentucky College of Dentistry*
*Lexington, KY 40536-0297, USA*
*E-mail address:* rhhaug2@uky.edu

ELSEVIER
SAUNDERS

Oral Maxillofacial Surg Clin N Am 17 (2005) xi – xii

ORAL AND
MAXILLOFACIAL
SURGERY CLINICS
of North America

Preface

# The Role of the Oral and Maxillofacial Surgeon in Wartime, Emergencies, and Terrorist Attacks

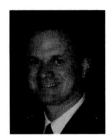

David B. Powers, DMD, MD
*Guest Editor*

Every generation of the American populace has a seminal event that defines their history and influences their outlook on life. When asked, people of each generation can tell you exactly where they were and what was occurring at the time of the event. For my grandparents' generation it was December 7, 1941—the shock of the attack on Pearl Harbor and the realization that World War II had begun for the United States. My parents related the impact of November 22, 1963, when President John F. Kennedy was assassinated, signaling the end to the so-called age of innocence and plunging the United States into an era of social and political turmoil that persisted throughout the remainder of the decade. For my generation, the event is obvious: September 11, 2001. It is not an exaggeration to say that life in the United States changed forever after that date. I vividly remember being at the AAOMS Meeting in Orlando, Florida, standing with approximately 100 people around a television watching the south tower of the World Trade Center collapse. Shock, disbelief, and confusion appeared to be the order of the day. After a few minutes I realized there was the potential for thousands of casualties that could overwhelm the local health care facilities, leaving many patients suffering needlessly awaiting care. The impetus for the creation of this issue of the *Oral and Maxillofacial Surgery Clinics of North America* came from that moment.

Since September 2001, the medical services of the armed forces of the United States have labored to provide the highest quality of care for our brave warriors injured during service to their country. Many lessons have been learned—and in some cases relearned—with regard to management of maxillofacial trauma. It is with great pride that I say my colleagues in the Army and Navy have worked with those of us in the Air Force to develop treatment protocols based on scientific criteria and clinical experience, helping our injured troops regain a quality of life they and their families felt may have been lost forever. During these experiences, our deployed oral and maxillofacial surgeons often found themselves having to provide a wide range of medical services because of the absolute inundation of the medical treatment facility with casualties. We realized this could easily occur in the United States with another terrorist attack or natural disaster, and felt a moral and ethical obligation to share our experiences with the civilian community. Although state and federal aid will eventually be mobilized and sent to the disaster location, local providers are often alone for the first 24 hours of any emergency situation. The goal of this issue is for civilian or military oral and maxillofacial surgeons to be able to take this book from their libraries and have a single source to assist them in the management of a wide assortment of casualties.

1042-3699/05/$ – see front matter. Published by Elsevier Inc.
doi:10.1016/j.coms.2005.04.006

I am thankful for an unbelievably supportive wife and loving family who have allowed me to undertake this task. I also would like to express my sincere appreciation to all of the authors for taking the time to share their expertise and clinical experiences. Finally, I dedicate this issue to the Marines, soldiers, sailors, and airmen of the United States Armed Forces, who display unbelievable bravery daily in the performance of their duties to their country; to their families, who are separated from loved ones far too often; to the injured warriors who have given me the honor to be involved in their care; and to those members of the military who have made the ultimate sacrifice in defense of the freedoms we all too often take for granted.

David B. Powers, DMD, MD
*59 MDW/MRDO*
*Department of Oral and Maxillofacial Surgery*
*2200 Bergquist Drive, Suite 1*
*Lackland Air Force Base, TX 78236-9908, USA*
*E-mail address:* david.powers@lackland.af.mil

ELSEVIER
SAUNDERS

Oral Maxillofacial Surg Clin N Am 17 (2005) 241 – 250

ORAL AND
MAXILLOFACIAL
SURGERY CLINICS
of North America

# Tissue Injury and Healing

Brent Kincaid, DDS[a],*, John P. Schmitz, DDS, PhD[b,c]

[a]Department of Oral and Maxillofacial Surgery, United States Air Force Academy, 10th Medical Group/SGDDH, USAFA,
4102 Pinion Drive, Colorado Springs, CO 80840, USA
[b]San Pedro Facial Surgery, 14500 San Pedro, Suite 102, San Antonio, TX 78232, USA
[c]Department of Orthopaedics, University of Texas Health Sciences Center, 7703 Floyd Curl Drive, San Antonio, TX 78229, USA

Wound healing is the vast branch of science that has a leg in medicine, biology, physiology, biochemistry, and art. It is perhaps one of the most studied processes in medicine—certainly in surgery—and yet until the last several decades, much of it remained a mystery. The large body of literature on wound healing has focused primarily on skin wounds, because they are the most common and easily studied wounds the human body can provide. Whether a surgical incision, simple traumatic laceration, or complex blast injury, the same basic pattern of repair exists in all wounds. The differentiating factors are the length of time spent in the various phases of wound healing. The modifying factors of foreign bodies, contamination, fragmentation, size of defect, associated thermal injury, and degree of functional impairment can alter critically the basic repair processes of the body. This article uses skin as the model to define acute wound healing and focuses on various types of wounding patterns expected to be seen in mass casualty scenarios. The article also includes discussion of adjuncts to wound healing and surgical reconstructive principles.

## Types of wound healing

There are two broad categories of wounds: acute and chronic. Chronic wounds never reach a functional endpoint and remain in the inflammatory phase of healing indefinitely. These types of wounds are not common in the maxillofacial region, mostly because of the abundant vascularity and relative ease of access to repair and clean. Acute wounds progress through all phases of the healing response and come to a functional endpoint. Acute wound repair attempts to establish this functional endpoint in as expedient a manner as possible and sacrifices the perfect regeneration of tissue in favor of quick restoration of anatomic barriers, blood flow, and tissue integrity [1,2].

Wounds heal or are repaired in one of three basic patterns: primary, delayed primary, and secondary. Primary closure is the most ordered and easily studied. The wound edges at the site of injury are reapproximated within hours of the insult, such as occurs with wound closure after a surgical procedure. Minimal contracture occurs in these types of wounds. With secondary closure, wound edges are left in their postinjury state and allowed to seal the wound by granulation and re-epithelialization followed by contraction. Closure by secondary intention is rarely needed in the maxillofacial region because of the abundant vascularity that aids the healing process, unlike any other cutaneous area of the body [2,3]. In the situation of significant avulsive injuries that require soft and hard tissue reconstruction, however, this approach may be the preferred method of repair. The surgeon must keep in mind that this technique ultimately must deal with the inherent scarring of large injuries, and this scarring is ultimately difficult—if not impossible—to overcome. Because scarring is increased in younger patients because of lack of excess tissue laxity, this is a particularly important

* Corresponding author.
*E-mail address:* bk2thman@yahoo.com (B. Kincaid).

1042-3699/05/$ – see front matter. Published by Elsevier Inc.
doi:10.1016/j.coms.2005.05.005

principle in handling war victims, who typically are in their late teens to early twenties. Delayed primary closure, or tertiary repair, eventually results in the reapproximation of tissue edges. First, however, it is treated by serial débridement to decrease the risk of infection and ensure that all nonviable tissue is excised. This is the typical way in which a large blast injury of the maxillofacial region is treated. As discussed later in this article, this technique and modifications thereof are increasingly being used in high-energy and avulsive wounds, particularly wounds in a mass casualty scenario.

**Phases of wound healing**

Various authors have divided the wound healing process into three, four, or five phases. For purposes of this discussion, the process is divided into three distinct phases, realizing that each phase is not a discrete event, but a correlated set of events along the complex continuum that is acute wound healing. These phases are hemostasis and inflammation, proliferation, and remodeling.

*Hemostasis and inflammation*

Upon disruption to the skin barrier, tiny blood vessels at the site of injury are disrupted and vasoconstriction occurs immediately because of the influence of thromboxane A-2 (locally) and epinephrine (systemically) [2–4]. Circulating platelets are exposed to tissue collagen and begin the well-described process of coagulation. As the platelets attach to collagen, they also begin adhering to other platelets, which forms a platelet plug. The coagulation cascade is set in motion and terminates in the formation of a fibrin plug, which further traps platelets and erythrocytes to produce a stable clot. In the physiologically normal host, this process occurs in seconds to minutes, depending on size and depth of injury.

As the clot is established and platelets are trapped, they are induced to release various bioactive proteins stored in $\alpha$-granules within the platelets. The $\alpha$-granules release platelet-derived growth factor (PDGF), transforming growth factor-$\beta$ (TGF-$\beta$), and fibroblast growth factor-2, among other cytokines [2–6]. These growth factors are important mediators of the inflammatory response and are active almost immediately after wounding takes place (Table 1). Their initial responsibility is to cause chemotaxis of neutrophils from the peripheral circulation to the site of injury.

Neutrophils are the first agents in the long cascade of leukocytes drawn to the wound area, and their activity is primary in the first 48 hours, although it is not entirely necessary. Studies have shown that the

Table 1
Selected cytokines in the wound healing process

| Cytokine | Cell source | Activity |
|---|---|---|
| PDGF | Platelets, macrophages, endothelial cells | Chemotaxis/activation of neutrophils, macrophages, fibroblasts, endothelial cells; involved in inflammation, angiogenesis, contraction, remodeling |
| TGF-$\alpha$ | Macrophages, lymphocytes, keratinocytes | Chemotaxis of neutrophils, fibroblast, and epithelial cell proliferation; involved in inflammation, angiogenesis, and epithelialization |
| TGF-$\beta$ | Platelets, lymphocytes, macrophages, endothelial cells, fibroblasts, keratinocytes | Chemotaxis of neutrophils, macrophages, lymphocytes, fibroblasts; involved in inflammation, angiogenesis, fibroplasias, and collagen synthesis |
| EGF | Platelets, macrophages | Fibroblast and epithelial cell proliferation |
| FGF | Macrophages, lymphocytes, endothelial cells, fibroblasts, mast cells | Fibroblast and epithelial cell proliferation; involved in angiogenesis, epithelialization, and remodeling |
| IGF | Macrophages, fibroblasts | Fibroblast proliferation and collagen synthesis, epithelial cell migration |
| VEGF | Keratinocytes | Increased vascular permeability, endothelial cell proliferation |
| TNF-$\alpha$ | Macrophages | Neutrophil degranulation, endothelial cell proliferation |
| IL-1 | Macrophages, keratinocytes | Vasodilation, pyrogenic, fibroblast proliferation, collagen synthesis, various immune functions |

*Abbreviations:* EGF, epidermal growth factor; FGF, fibroblast growth factor; IGF, insulin-like growth factor; IL, interleukin; PDGF, platelet-derived growth factor; TGF, tissue growth factor; TNF, tumor necrosis factor; VEGF, vascular endothelial growth factor.

absence of neutrophils does not prevent healing, but their presence in the early stages of wounds jump starts the process and is important for the speed and efficiency of the system [1,4,6]. When present, they function as scavengers and remove bacteria, damaged tissue, and foreign debris. Circulating neutrophils slow down and rim the endothelial lining of vessels during margination through carefully coordinated signals via tumor necrosis factor-α) and interleukin-1. Thus slowed, they enter the wound area by migrating through the permeable endothelial cells in the process of diapedesis. This increase in vascular permeability is mediated in part by serotonin released from the dense bodies of platelets [2,7]. At that point, the early vasoconstriction, which is designed to limit initial injury, has given way to vasodilation to increase the rate of delivery of inflammatory cells. The result of this shift is the well-known inflammation quartet of rubor (redness caused by vasodilation secondary to prostacyclin and prostaglandin activity), tumor (edema caused by increased blood flow and extravasation of plasma proteins), calor (warmth caused by increased blood flow and local metabolism), and dolor (pain caused by edema and the action of various prostaglandins).

As the neutrophil response begins to wane after 24 to 48 hours, cell predominance shifts to the macrophage, which is an essential cell for the healing process. Macrophages are cells that evolve from fixed tissue monocytes and are attracted to the wounded area by numerous cytokines [3,8,9], including PDGF and TGF-β released by the platelets shortly after wounding. These cells are primarily responsible for wound débridement via phagocytosis, release of nitric oxide (antimicrobial function), and extracellular matrix degradation and synthesis [6]. Perhaps more importantly, macrophages release additional growth factors responsible for a wide range of activities, from chemotaxis to proliferation of various cell types involved in the next (proliferative) phase of healing. Among the cytokines released by macrophages are interleukin-1, which is well known for its pyrogenic role in addition to promoting vasodilation, enhancing fibroblast proliferation, and performing important immune regulatory functions; additional PDGF for fibroblast chemotaxis; TGF-β, which is critical in angiogenesis and collagen deposition; and tumor necrosis factor-α, which assists endothelial cell proliferation [10].

## Proliferation

The initial response to wounding concentrates on limiting damage and débriding the wound of bacterial

invasion. As these processes stabilize the wound in the first 48 hours, the inflammatory component of healing begins to wane and there is a gradual shift toward reconstituting tissue via fibroblast proliferation and angiogenesis. One of the two primary cell lines in this process is the fibroblast, which is recruited to the area via fibroblast growth factor, PDGF, TGF-B, epidermal growth factor, and insulin-like growth factor-1. Fibroblasts that enter the wound area are derived from differentiation of local mesenchymal cells and activation of quiescent fibroblasts rather than margination from ingrowing vascular supply [11]. Macrophage-released cytokines are responsible for these changes and the stimulus to begin collagen deposition. This process, typically active by day 5, is responsible for the lag time while inflammation decreases (48 hours) and before actual fibroplasia takes place [2]. This collagen matrix formation is in the active phase for up to 2 to 3 weeks, when the deposition and breakdown equilibrates and the remodeling or maturation phase is entered. The initial matrix that is established in this phase is expedient but not orderly, and it lacks strength. Along with collagen deposition, specialized cells called myofibroblasts migrate into the area and cause wound contraction, a protective mechanism that decreases the size of the wound and attempts to provide protection to the wound bed. Once this process is complete, usually within 3 weeks, myofibroblasts leave the area [8].

The second key component of the proliferative phase is the process of angiogenesis, which typically begins after 48 hours and is complete by 2 weeks. The scaffold of vascular growth into the wound is provided by endothelial cells, which are attracted to the area by fibroblast growth factor, PDGF, specifically vascular endothelial growth factor, tumor necrosis factor-α, and TGF-β. These cytokines are primarily derived from platelets within the established fibrin clot and local macrophages. Tissue hypoxia and the creation of an oxygen gradient is chemoattractive for capillary growth [4]. Eventually, these capillary buds anastomose with each other and form extensive vascular loops within the wound, which allows the proliferative phase, and later remodeling, to progress quickly [12].

The final component of the proliferative phase is epithelialization. If a wound has been closed primarily, migrating epithelial cells typically bridge the microscopic gap between wound edges within 24 to 48 hours. Wounds with partial-thickness injury must epithelialize across a much larger gap, however, which is accomplished by epithelial cell proliferation from the wound edges and from adnexal structures that remain in the wound bed. The free epithelial edges, along with potent cytokines, are responsible for initiating the cells to migrate and proliferate. This process, described as tumbling over each other, continues until cell-to-cell contact is made across the wound gap, at which time contact inhibition causes the cells to cease proliferation [3,8]. As the epithelial cells are establishing a migrating sheet over the wound bed, their basement membrane and intercellular bridging is reformed, which provides a renewed barrier [13].

*Remodeling*

As the wound healing process enters the third week, net collagen deposition begins to slow. At that point the amount of collagen present in the wound has peaked in quantity but is still poorly organized, and the wound provides only 15% the strength of intact, uninjured skin [8]. Remodeling is accomplished by a dynamic process of collagen breakdown and new collagen synthesis that is essentially in equilibrium but results in removal of the initial, thin, unorganized fibers with replacement by thicker, highly crossed-linked fibers oriented along directional stress lines of the wound [13]. By 6 weeks, the wound has achieved 50% to 60% of final end strength through this fiber reorientation. Maximal strength occurs by 6 months but still is less than 80% of intact skin strength. Although this remodeling phase can continue for up to 1 year, the overall strength of the scar tissue does not continue to improve after 6 months. If proliferation continues through the remodeling phase and beyond, hypertrophic scars or keloids develop.

## Wounding mechanisms

Because war has become more complex and less defined, many oral and maxillofacial surgeons one day will face the challenges of helping to care for victims of terrorism, perhaps in a mass casualty scenario. It is important to understand the modern changing wound patterns. Injury patterns and complications from the ongoing conflicts in Iraq and Afghanistan can teach us a great deal about their treatment. These injuries are not the sole responsibility of the military surgeon, however. The World Trade Center attacks of September 11, 2001, the Atlanta Olympic Village attack in 1996, the Oklahoma City bombing of 1995, and the World Trade Center bombing of 1993 were significant recent events performed on American soil that required

the excellent response of civilian providers to deal with these mass casualty scenarios. By studying these events and others like them around the world, injury can be better anticipated, understood, and treated, ultimately resulting in decreased mortality and morbidity.

Wounding occurs from physical (mechanical) forces that cause characteristic injury patterns. Wounding can occur from explosive blasts, gunshot wounds, shotgun wounds, sharp objects, blunt forces, and other forces. Each of these forces interacts with tissues and causes distinct wound characteristics. As more experience is gained and more is learned about these wounds, treatment can be tailored better to affect an optimum outcome. Much of what we have learned historically from treating various types of wounds in large metropolitan trauma centers, however, is being revised based on new models of injury, infection, and healing of soldiers and civilians involved in the current conflicts in Iraq and Afghanistan. The author (BLK) has noted significant problems of late, including unusual infections, antibiotic resistance, and significant early scarring that impairs the wound healing process and challenges the treatment planning of the reconstructive surgeon. Although recent protocols have suggested delayed immediate repair to take advantage of the primary phases of wound healing, often atypical bacterial strains remain seeded and unaffected by usual first-line antibiotic treatment. When early reconstruction is performed, the results may be compromised by a high rate of late, antibiotic-resistant infections. When reconstruction is delayed to ensure clean wounds, significant scarring debilitates the reconstructive efforts. We are presented with the reconstructive paradox. Early repair avoids scar contracture but is more susceptible to late infection and compromise of the repair; late repair ensures a clean, segregated wound bed but faces the irreversible effects of contracture.

## Analysis of wounds using a mechanical theory of injury

Wounds to skin and the underlying bone occur through various biomechanical forces. Analysis of the cause of injury (eg, striking a steering wheel, falling on a stairs, dog bite) is vital to planning the surgical repair. Surface injury, just as bone fractures, can be classified before repair. Surface injury occurs from shear, tension, and compression. The mechanical injury determines the surgical approach.

## Lacerations

Lacerations of the skin may be caused by sharp objects striking the skin (eg, knives, glass). These injuries are developed by a shearing effect on the skin. Because little energy is imparted to the skin by sharp objects, minimal adjacent injury is created. These wounds have a low incidence of infection and usually heal with acceptable scarring.

Tension injuries occur as the result of an object hitting the skin (Fig. 1). These injuries commonly occur from angulated objects (eg, steering wheels, stairs) striking the skin at an oblique angle. Blood vessels and the skin adjacent to the wound edge are stretched and torn. Devitalized skin is often present adjacent to the wound margin, and when these angled injuries occur, the wound margins are frequently beveled. Correction of beveled wound margins by creating an edge perpendicular to the surface enhances repair by better aligning the wound edges and creating a more aesthetic scar.

Compression injuries occur when blunt, rounded objects (eg, rocks, baseball bats) strike the skin either perpendicular to or at angles to the skin. The skin is often ragged and ecchymosis is present. Significant devitalized skin and muscle may be present but may not declare themselves for several days. These wounds are more susceptible to infection and require pressure lavage irrigation (Pulsavac; Zimmer, Inc., Warsaw, Indiana) to assist in débridement, encourage granulation tissue, and aid in removal of necrotic tissue. These wounds may have to be treated in a delayed fashion, often after serial sessions of débridement or wet-to-dry dressing changes.

## Blast injury

The modern terrorist event increasingly involves explosives, specifically improvised explosive devices. The resulting injuries are often different from motor vehicle collisions, interpersonal violence, or industrial accidents that are typical in a level I trauma center. To understand the effects of blast injuries, it is necessary first to understand the nature of the explosion. There are multiple forces at work after the detonation of an explosive device. The primary blast wave is a wave of positive pressure that emanates from the explosion and causes a compression of the surrounding air, which results in the creation of rapid overpressure that spreads circumferentially. The amplitude of this overpressure wave is one of the primary determinants of survivability, along with impulse, or the duration of the peak wave. High-velocity explosives, such as ammonium nitrate and fuel oil and C4, cause shattering or brisance [14]. Low-velocity explosives, such as ordinary gunpowder, cause pushing forces rather than shatter. After this overpressure wave is a second phase, known as a negative pressure wave. This wave occurs as the surrounding atmosphere rushes to fill the displacement caused by the positive pressure first phase. As this wave propagates, it draws surrounding debris

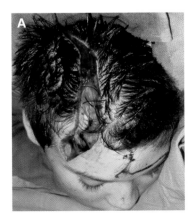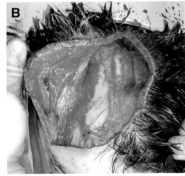

Fig. 1. Degloving facial laceration. The patient was a restrained front seat passenger in a T-bone motor vehicle collision. In this high-speed crash, his head contacted the front windshield, a flat fixed object, which caused a tearing injury. The laceration appeared straight line and simple on initial examination (A), but on exploration under general anesthesia, it found to deglove superficial to the temporalis muscle and extend to the right base of the ear (B). Microscopically the wound margins (and collagen of the extracellular matrix) have been stretched, as has the microvessel architecture of the wound margin.

into its wake, which is responsible for many of the secondary injuries seen [14–16].

Blast injuries are generally described as primary, secondary, and tertiary. The primary blast injury is caused by the first phase overpressure wave and affects air-filled organs (ie, ears, lungs, bowels, central nervous system). Not only does this wave cause rupture but also it can cause shear-type injuries as tissues of different densities (bone, blood vessels, brain) react to the pressure change [16]. The primary blast injury is responsible for most immediate deaths related to blast injury. Initial assessment and débridement of wounds may account for direct tissue injury, but late tissue ischemia often occurs, which increases the area of necrosis as the effects of shear injury on vascular tissues gradually decline.

The secondary blast injury is caused by surrounding debris and shrapnel that is within the explosive device being propelled or drawn into the victim, which results in penetrating injury patterns. The debris may include shattered bomb casings, glass from surrounding structures, shrapnel placed in the explosive, or—increasingly in the case of terrorists and suicide bombers—human tissue. This human tissue is deliberately placed in explosive devices and is aimed at increasing contamination of victims. The secondary blast injuries may be mild, moderate, or severe, depending on the type and depth of penetration. In wartime scenarios, these injuries are more likely to occur in the maxillofacial region and extremities because of Kevlar shielding and other protective military garments, which have proved efficacious in protecting the core. Although current statistics are unavailable, the last century of warfare has shown that the American soldier consistently suffers 10% to 20% of penetrating injuries to the head and neck region [17]. In the civilian setting, penetrating injuries are likely to be present in individuals who survive hospital triage.

Tertiary blast injury occurs as a result of bodily displacement of a victim incidental to the blast wave. These injuries present similarly to other blunt force trauma and often involve fractures of the maxillofacial complex. In victims of explosion, there should be high suspicion for penetrating and blunt injury patterns in survivors, who are treated according to their injury pattern, as would typically occur in a civilian trauma center [18]. One of the newer challenges facing surgeons responsible for repair and reconstruction of these victims involves the increasingly diverse infections present in these wounds. Human tissue incorporated into a blast device easily can seed atypical bacteria deep into a wound bed—bacteria that may not be susceptible to

standard first-line antibiotics aimed at skin or oral flora.Hum These injuries may require delayed primary closure with serial débridement and aggressive antibiotic therapy to ensure a clean wound. As discussed later in this article, wound infection is one of the complicating factors increasingly seen in these types of wounds. Some surgeons have advocated avoidance of primary closure of blast wounds [19], although the abundant vascularity of the maxillofacial region allows greater latitude with closure than found elsewhere in the body. Basic principles of wound management still must be followed, however. Contaminated wounds can be converted to surgically clean wounds if treated early with débridement and irrigation, but infected wounds—those with signs of inflammation—cannot [20]. Whereas studies have shown that bacterial counts in wounds can reach critical level within 6 hours [21] and double within 12 hours of injury, time is not the sole factor responsible for wound infection. Type of inoculum, depth of penetration, local host defenses, and interval treatment are important modifiers of the degree of infection that develops.

## Gunshot wounds

The available literature on firearm injuries is voluminous, much of which is flat out incorrect or controversial at best. Elsewhere in this issue, many of these myths are dispelled. For the purposes of tissue injury and treatment paradigms as related to firearm injuries, it is important to understand the wounding mechanisms.

Fackler [22–24] has contributed greatly to correcting many of the widely held myths in the medical and surgical literature with a series of papers. Inordinate attention has been given to injury classification based solely on projectile velocity, citing low-velocity (<2000 ft/s), high-velocity (2000–4500 ft/s), and ultra–high-velocity (>4500 ft/s) projectiles as key determinants in injury pattern [25]. Scientific study and practical experience on the battlefield and in emergency rooms have taught that more important factors include projectile type (ie, jacketed versus nonjacketed), shape, victim proximity to muzzle (shotgun injuries), body armor that may have been penetrated, and the specific tissues encountered [22–24, 26,27]. For example, unlike the abdomen, pelvis, or many extremity wounds, the maxillofacial region consists of a highly osseous framework with a relatively thin soft tissue drape. The influence of bone fragmentation and secondary missiles is far more prevalent in this region and significantly impacts wounding and treatment.

Numerous authors have proclaimed "treat the wound, not the weapon." By following this rationale, appropriate surgical treatment principles are adhered to and the wound is individually treated based on presentation and mechanism, rather than an arbitrary adherence to an unsubstantiated classification system. As such, wounds can be viewed as penetrating, perforating, or avulsive and managed according to the resultant injuries [25]. In penetrating wounds, the projectile remains within the target and typically causes soft tissue laceration and possibly bony fracture as all the kinetic energy is transferred to the victim. These injuries should be handled in the manner in which typical blunt trauma injury is treated: direct open approaches to expose the fractures and débridement of injured soft tissue followed by reduction, rigid internal fixation, and primary soft tissue closure. Similarly, in perforating injuries the projectile exits the tissue and leaves an entrance and exit wound, which should be managed as described for penetrating injuries.

Avulsive wounds demonstrate significant loss of soft or hard tissue and are typically the result of high-energy projectiles (high-velocity rifle or close-range shotgun). Historically, these wounds have a higher incidence of complications (ie, infection, comminution, non-union, and residual cosmetic and functional deformities) that can be more difficult to manage. Typically these injuries require multiple operative interventions and true craniofacial principles to reestablish vertical and horizontal facial pillars and anterior projection. Because variable amounts of tissue are lost, primary or secondary grafting is required to replace soft and hard tissue bulk (Fig. 3). In many of the victims treated in the United States from the current theater of operations in Iraq and Afghanistan, the extent of fibrosis and scarring is a more significant factor than previously seen, mostly because of the evolving types of weapons being used in terrorist attacks.

Two main treatment protocols exist for these types of wounds. An excellent protocol for management of avulsive injuries to the maxillofacial region has been described by Clark and colleagues [28] and Robertson and Manson [29,30]. This protocol may be termed the immediate bone soft tissue protocol. Briefly, those authors advocate that any high-energy or avulsive injury of the maxillofacial region be approached with a systematic algorithm as follows: (1) initial débridement and excision of necrotic tissue followed by soft tissue closure and intravenous antibiotic therapy, (2) repair of bone injury with traditional open reduction and fixation techniques used for blunt facial injuries, (3) serial débridement every 24 to 48 hours, which involves reopening the soft tissues in the area of avulsion and further débriding interval necrotic tissue, hematoma, infection, and dead space, followed by closure of the soft tissue wound, and (4) definitive reconstruction with pedicled or free-tissue transfer to replace bone and soft tissue loss when the wound is stable.

Conservative débridement initially is performed to minimize the amount of viable tissue that is excised on first look, yet it ensures through serial débridement that all necrotic tissue is eventually removed as it declares. By performing definitive reconstruction early (within the first 2 weeks is recommended), the surgeon is able to take advantage of the primary phase of wound healing and optimally can avoid the detrimental effects of scars and wound contracture that are nearly impossible to overcome. The disadvantage of this protocol is that the surgeon must ensure that the wound bed is free of infection and necrotic tissue before grafting, because these factors could compromise the graft.

Others advocate a secondary reconstruction (delayed soft tissue bone graft) by achieving soft tissue closure with serial débridement as needed and then returning in 3 months after intraoral mucosal closure and maturation are achieved and performing bone grafting via autogenous rib, cranium, ilium, or vascularized free-tissue transfer [25]. The advantages with this technique are that the surgeon can ensure a healthy graft bed that is partitioned from oral contamination at the time of graft placement and a patient's healing mechanisms can be optimized in terms of nutrition, bacterial elimination, and possible revascularization through hyperbaric oxygen treatment. Maximal time is allowed for the intensive preoperative planning that may be required, including obtaining radiologic images or stereolithographic models. The obvious disadvantage is that the effects of fibrosis and scar contracture are irreversible and are difficult to overcome via secondary procedure.

A protocol that averts many of the disadvantages of the prior approaches is one advocated by one the coauthors (JPS). It may be considered an immediate combined approach. In this protocol, intravenous antibiotics are instituted immediately, and after initial patient stabilization, the wound is irrigated using a Pulse-Evac and débrided to remove all gross debris and identify vascular wound edges. Presuturing is used to decrease the size of avulsive wounds and prepare the wound bed for definitive reconstruction. A complete reconstructive approach is executed using full-thickness cranial bone or fibular free flaps to

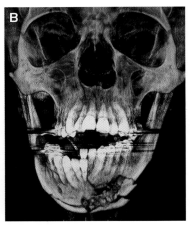

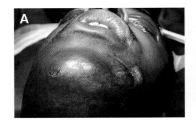

Fig. 2. Penetrating handgun injury. The patient suffered a mandibular injury as the victim of a drive-by shooting. The weapon was a handgun (low velocity), entrance and exit wounds (penetrating) were present in the lower face and left upper extremity. (*A*) Initial examination showed small, minimally destructive, soft tissue injury. (*B*) Radiographic studies later showed the significant degree of bony comminution not readily apparent on first glance. The surgeon should have high suspicion for significant bony defects with firearms injuries, despite outward appearances.

reconstruct the facial skeleton. Local, regional, or free flaps are used to close all tissue defects.

### Shotgun wounds

Unlike other firearm injuries that are often described in terms of muzzle velocity, shotgun wounds are typically classified a different way. Whereas shotguns always produce low-velocity projectiles, they are clustered as numerous small pellets capable of deformation, and their cumulative effect often can be more devastating than higher energy projectiles (Fig. 2). As they travel farther from the muzzle, they disperse in the air and the composite effect of their energy quickly dissipates. Shotgun injuries are classified according to the distance between the muzzle and the target, or alternatively according to pellet scatter, because injury history may not be reliable. Both systems grade three types of injury, with type I being the least severe and type III the most severe. Type I injuries are those in which the distance from muzzle to victim is more than 7 yards, type II sets the distance between 3 and 7 yards, and type III marks the distance as less than 3 yards [31,32]. The farther from the muzzle the target is hit, the more dispersed are the pellets and the greater decrease in velocity has occurred. Type I injuries are also associated with more than 25 $cm^2$ area between the extremes of pellet scatter, type II has an area of 10 $cm^2$ to 25 $cm^2$, and type III has an area less than

10 $cm^2$ [31]. The more severe shotgun injuries (type II and III) are similar to the high-energy, avulsive type injuries previously described (Fig. 4). These wounds often result in significant tissue loss and more severe destruction than is readily apparent from superficial wounds. In contrast, type I shotgun injuries are more similar to low-energy projectile wounds, with often just superficial soft tissue disruption or simple hard tissue injury that resembles low-impact blunt trauma. These different types of

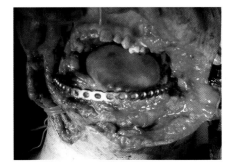

Fig. 3. Avulsive blast injury. The patient suffered significant avulsive hard and soft tissue injury after being the victim of an improvised explosive device while deployed in Iraq during Operation Iraqi Freedom. He lost a significant portion of mandible from angle to angle and the associated facial soft tissues. After serial débridement, he was treated initially with reconstruction bar and latissimus dorsi microvascular free tissue transfer and staged secondary bone graft.

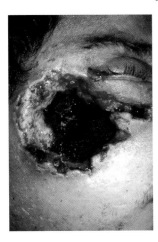

Fig. 4. Shotgun wound to right face. The patient received a shotgun wound to the right face at point-blank range. A large area of tissue avulsion is present. Of note are the irregular wound edges and gross evidence of devitalized tissue. Areas of vital tissue must be delineated before beginning reconstruction. The patient was taken to the operating room on multiple occasions for Pulse-Evac irrigation of the wound edges and presuturing to decrease the size of the defect. The defect eventually was closed with a temporalis flap and the facial skeleton was stabilized with cranial bone.

shotgun injuries are treated in accordance with their wounding pattern rather than their source weapon.

## Other wounding mechanisms

Other confounding wound factors that may alter significantly the management protocol include involvement of nuclear, biologic, or chemical weapons (so-called "weapons of mass destruction") and burn injuries, which often accompany blast victims. These modifiers are discussed elsewhere in this issue.

## Summary

We have attempted to provide a primer on the biochemistry of wound healing for clinical oral and maxillofacial surgeons, recognizing that time frames, tissue growth, and cell types are important factors in the healing process that may influence treatment, whereas the specifics of molecular composition and fiber interaction are less critical at the tissue level. Various injury patterns, including different types of lacerations, blunt and penetrating trauma, blast injuries, and ballistic injuries, have been described with an eye toward the ultimate clinical goals of

functional and cosmetic reconstruction. As injuries of our incredibly brave military soldiers are studied and treated and their outcomes ultimately assessed, they serve as the models to help us understand changing wound patterns and effects in this new age of terroristic warfare. It is our duty as surgeons to take these lessons, modify our protocols where indicated, incorporate this newfound knowledge in our practice, and ultimately pass on this critical corporate knowledge so that military and civilian surgeons alike can be prepared in the future for whatever mass casualty scenarios may present.

## References

[1] Glat PM, Longaker MT. Wound healing. In: Grabb and Smith's plastic surgery. 5th edition. Philadelphia: Lippincott-Raven; 1997. p. 3–12

[2] Leong M, Phillips LG. Wound healing. In: Townsend CM, Beauchamp RD, Evers BM, et al, editors. Sabiston textbook of surgery: the biologic basis of modern surgical practice. 17th edition. Philadelphia: W.B. Saunders; 2004. p. 183–207.

[3] Monaco JL, Lawrence WT. Acute wound healing: an overview. Clin Plast Surg 2003;30:1–12.

[4] Steed DL. The role of growth factors in wound healing. Surg Clin North Am 1997;77:575–86.

[5] Krizek TJ, Harries RHC, Robson MC. Biology of tissue injury and repair. In: Georgiade GS, Riefkohl R, Levin LS, editors. Plastic, maxillofacial, and reconstructive surgery. 3rd edition. Baltimore: Lippincott, Williams and Wilkins; 1999. p. 3–9.

[6] Witte MB, Barbul A. General principles of wound healing. Surg Clin North Am 1997;77:509–28.

[7] Kloth LC, McCulloch JM. The inflammatory response to wounding. In: McCulloch JM, Kloth LC, Feedar JA, editors. Wound healing: alternatives in management. 2nd edition. Philadelphia: F.A. Davis Company; 1995. p. 3–15.

[8] Lawrence WT. Physiology of the acute wound. Clin Plast Surg 1998;25:321–39.

[9] Giglio JA, Abubaker AO, Diegelmann RF. Physiology of wound healing of skin and mucosa. Oral Maxillofacial Surg Clin N Am 1996;8:457–65.

[10] Wahl LM, Wahl SM. Inflammation. In: Cohen IK, Diegelmann RF, Lindblad WJ, editors. Wound healing: biochemical and clinical aspects. Philadelphia: W.B. Saunders; 1992. p. 40–62.

[11] Morgan CJ, Pledger WJ, Fibroblast proliferation. In: Cohen IK, Diegelmann RF, Lindblad WJ, editors. Wound healing: biochemical and clinical aspects. Philadelphia: W.B. Saunders; 1992. p. 63-76.

[12] Whalen GF, Zetter BR. Angiogenesis. In: Cohen IK, Diegelmann RF, Lindblad WJ, editors. Wound healing: biochemical and clinical aspects. Philadelphia: W.B. Saunders; 1992. p. 77–95.

[13] Stucki-McCormick SU, Santiago PE. The metabolic and physiologic aspects of wound healing. Oral Maxillofacial Surg Clin N Am 1996;8:467–76.

[14] Lacombe DM, Miller GT, Dennis JD. Primary blast injury: an EMS guide to pathophysiology, assessment and management. JEMS 2004;71:86–9.

[15] Singer P, Cohen JD, Stein M. Conventional terrorism and critical care. Crit Care Med 2005;33(Suppl): S61–5.

[16] Wang Z, Liu Y, Lei D, et al. A new model of blast injury from a spherical explosive and its special wound in the maxillofacial region. Mil Med 2003; 168:330–2.

[17] Borden Institute. Weapons effects and parachute injuries. In: Szul AC, Davis LB, editors. Emergency war surgery. Third United States Revision. Washington, DC: Borden Institute; 2004. p. 1.1–1.2.

[18] Antonyshyn O, Gruss JS. Complex facial trauma. In: McMurtry RY, McLellan BA, editor. Management of blunt trauma. Baltimore: Williams and Wilkins; 1990. p. 359–90.

[19] Langworthy MJ, Sabra J, Gould M. Terrorism and blast phenomena: lessons learned from the attack on the USS Cole. Clin Orthop 2004;422:82–7.

[20] Peacock EE. Wound repair. 3rd edition. Philadelphia: W.B. Saunders; 1984. p. 141–86, 485–503.

[21] Cunningham LL, Haug RH, Ford J. Firearm injuries to the maxillofacial region: an overview of current thoughts regarding demographics, pathophysiology, and management. J Oral Maxillofac Surg 2003;61: 932–42.

[22] Fackler ML, Bellamy RF, Malinowsky JA. A reconsideration of the wounding mechanism of very high-velocity projectiles: importance of projectile shape. J Trauma 1998;28:S63–7.

[23] Fackler ML. Gunshot wound review. Ann Emerg Med 1996;28:194–203.

[24] Fackler ML. Civilian gunshot wounds and ballistics: dispelling the myths. Emerg Med Clin North Am 1998;16:17–28.

[25] Osbourne TE, Bays RA. Pathophysiology and management of gunshot wounds to the face. In: Fonseca RJ, Walker RV, editors. Oral and maxillofacial trauma. 2nd edition. Philadelphia: W.B. Saunders; 1997. p. 948–81.

[26] Santucci RA, Chang Y. Ballistics for physicians: myths about wound ballistics and gunshot injuries. J Urol 2004;171:1408–14.

[27] Bartlett CS. Clinical update: gunshot wound ballistics. Clin Orthop Relat Res 2003;408:28–57.

[28] Clark N, Birely B, Manson PN, et al. High-energy ballistic and avulsive facial injuries: classification, patterns, and an algorithm for primary reconstruction. Plast Reconstr Surg 1996;98:585–601.

[29] Robertson B, Manson PN. The importance of serial débridement and "second-look" procedures in high-energy ballistic and avulsive facial injuries. Operative Techniques in Plastic and Reconstructive Surgery 1998;5:236–45.

[30] Robertson BC, Manson PN. High-energy ballistic and avulsive injuries: a management protocol for the next millennium. Surg Clin North Am 1999;79: 1489–502.

[31] Haug RH. Gunshot wounds to the head and neck. In: Kelly JPW, editor. Oral and maxillofacial surgery knowledge update. Chicago: American Association of Oral and Maxillofacial Surgeons; 1995. p. 65–82.

[32] Bartlett CS. Clinical update: gunshot wound ballistics. Clin Orthop Relat Res 2003;408:28–57.

ELSEVIER
SAUNDERS

Oral Maxillofacial Surg Clin N Am 17 (2005) 251 – 259

**ORAL AND
MAXILLOFACIAL
SURGERY CLINICS**
of North America

# Ten Common Myths of Ballistic Injuries

## David B. Powers, DMD, MD*, O. Bailey Robertson, DDS

*Department of Oral and Maxillofacial Surgery, Wilford Hall Medical Center, 2200 Bergquist Drive, Suite 1,
Lackland Air Force Base, San Antonio, TX 78236-9908, USA*

Handling ballistic injuries to the head and neck region unfortunately is a common occurrence for oral and maxillofacial surgeons. The recent conflicts in Iraq and Afghanistan have forced military surgeons to question the validity of many of the principles of treatment to which we were exposed during the course of our training. The basis of any discussion of ballistic injuries is recognizing the two mechanisms by which projectiles cause tissue damage: crushing and stretching. Any investigation of ballistic injuries after 1970 is in some way based on the work of Martin Fackler, from the International Wound Ballistics Association, who is generally considered to have brought true scientific, critical evaluation to the study of ballistics [1–13]. Santucci and Chang [14] performed a comprehensive review of the literature in 2004 of all documented articles relating to ballistic injuries and published their findings of four common myths regarding treatment of gunshot injuries. Whereas this article notes four common myths regarding the treatment of ballistic injuries, our clinical experience and recently gathered data published in the third edition of "Emergency War Surgery" produce additional areas of confusion

[15]. This article discusses ten common myths improperly perpetuated in the area of oral and maxillofacial surgery.

## Myth 1: The caliber of the projectile is important information for the management of a patient

Rifles, handguns, and submachine guns have rifled barrels—essentially, spiral grooves cut into the length of the interior of the bore of the barrel (Fig. 1) [16]. The grooves are separated by segments of metal, called lands, which project into the middle of the barrel. The diameter of the barrel measured between the lands represents the caliber of the projectile. Caliber specifications based on nomenclature used in the United States are confusing. The .30-06 and the Winchester .308 cartridges are both loaded with bullets that have a diameter of .308 inches [16]. The "06" in this term describes the year, 1906, when the cartridge was introduced to the market. The term "grains" originally was applied to black powder charges and refers to the weight of the powder in the cartridge, not the number of granules contained in the cartridge case. A .30-30 cartridge has a .308-inch diameter bullet propelled by 30 grains of smokeless powder [16]. As newer forms of gunpowder were developed, this powder charge was no longer used, but the terminology persists. Additional confusion exists because North Atlantic Treaty Organization (NATO) and United States military projectiles are described using the metric system. Although the question commonly is asked by medical personnel in

The views presented in this article reflect those of the authors and do not represent the official policies of the United States Air Force, the Department of Defense, or any branches of the United States government.

\* Corresponding author.

*E-mail address:* David.Powers@Lackland.af.mil (D.B. Powers).

1042-3699/05/$ – see front matter. Published by Elsevier Inc.
doi:10.1016/j.coms.2005.05.001

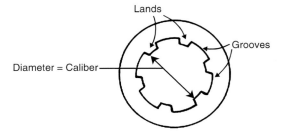

Fig. 1. Cross-section of a rifled barrel indicating the caliber of the weapon, which is measured as the distance between the lands.

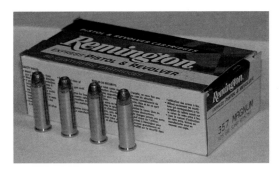

Fig. 3. .357 Magnum ammunition. Note longer shell case, which contains an increased amount of gunpowder charge but otherwise has a similar shape of projectile.

the initial resuscitation of a patient, the caliber of the projectile essentially makes no real difference in the treatment of a patient.

## Myth 2: Magnum cartridges shoot different ammunition and cause more serious injuries

To understand the fallacy of this concept, a detailed examination the .38 Special and .357 Magnum cartridges must be undertaken. Weapons designed for these projectiles essentially have identical internal bore dimensions when measured from the lands of the barrel. The .357 Magnum handgun is able to chamber and fire .38 Special ammunition (Fig. 2), but the reverse situation is not possible. The reason for this is that the .357 Magnum cartridge (Fig. 3) basically is the .38 Special cartridge with the case lengthened and additional propellant added to increase the velocity of the projectile [16]. The sole purpose of the larger Magnum charge is to produce a higher velocity bullet; the characteristics of the projectile are otherwise similar to conventional cartridges. Magnum shotgun ammunition may or may not be a physically larger cartridge and it

definitely has more propellant, but it does not contain more shot than the standard shell. The surgical care and management of injuries sustained by Magnum ammunition and conventional ammunition is similar. The higher velocity of the Magnum projectile does not translate into increased severity of wounds, but it does increase the effective range of the load [2,14,17].

## Myth 3: High-velocity projectiles cause greater injury and more traumatic wounding than low-velocity projectiles

The terms "high velocity" and "low velocity" as they relate to projectiles can be somewhat confusing. Consensus between US and European research does not occur in the literature, with varying definitions correlating to where the study was performed. The US literature designates high velocity as being between 2000 and 3000 ft/s (610–914 m/s), whereas studies from the United Kingdom designate the line between low and high velocity projectiles as being 1100 ft/s (335 m/s), which is the speed of sound in air [2]. The earliest recognized entry of high-velocity projectiles having an association with increased wounding potential occurred during the Vietnam War. In 1967, Rich reported in the *Journal of the American Medical Association* that bullets fired from the M16 rifle inflicted tremendous tissue destruction and injuries upon enemy combatants [17]. The muzzle velocity of the projectile shot from the M16 was 3100 ft/s. When coupled with erroneous information published by Rybeck in 1974 and in the 1975 edition of the "Emergency War Surgery" manual regarding the size of the temporary cavity caused by the missile, this information led to the

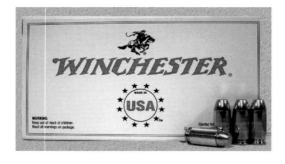

Fig. 2. .38 Special ammunition.

common misperception that high-velocity projectiles caused more significant injuries [2,18].

Part of the confusion regarding the wounding potential of high-velocity projectiles is caused by misinterpretation of ballistic gelatin model studies. Ballistic gelatin is 10% to 20% gelatin refrigerated to 4 to 10°C and is used as the tissue model for ballistic studies [8,14]. The wound profile diagrams included in this article and others represent the findings of these studies. The validity of the ballistic gelatin model has been confirmed by comparison with human autopsies, although there is confusion in correlating these studies to living patients, because the human body is much more resistant to deformation than gelatin [1,3,14,19]. The effects of skin resistance, clothing, and resistance to separation of the fascial planes cannot be replicated in gelatin. Harvey and colleagues [20] evaluated the two types of pressure waves produced by penetrating objects in 1947: the sonic pressure wave and the temporary cavity [2]. The first wave is the sonic pressure wave, sometimes referred to as the "shock wave," and it relates the sound of the projectile striking the target. This wave transmits at the speed of sound (ie, approximately 4750 ft/s [1450 m/s]) and is traveling considerably faster than the projectile entering the target [2]. No temporary cavity is formed with the sonic pressure wave, and in that regard it is analogous to the lithotripsy devices used for renal calculi destruction, with corresponding minimal risks for tissue injury [15]. Although American and Swedish researchers have tried to disprove Harvey's conclusions, no definitive evidence suggests that his findings are in error, and additional studies by French and American researchers support the original findings of 1947 [2,4,7,21–25]. The secondary pressure wave, referred to as the temporary cavity, is formed when the penetrating projectile strikes tissue and the wave radiates away laterally. After being struck by the projectile, the ballistic gelatin/tissue displays an obvious temporary cavity, which potentially injures tissues such as muscle, vessels, and organs. The clinical significance of this cavity is variable with no real consensus in the literature, and the temporary cavity caused by the M16 in animal laboratory models is much smaller than the approximate 18-cm temporary cavity seen in ballistic gelatin [14]. Dog models indicated that acute tissue injury secondary to temporary cavity formation sustained with high-velocity projectile strikes were no more than 5 cm and were able to resolve within 72 hours [14,26,27].

The United States military conducted extensive research into the wounding patterns of projectiles, and the results are summarized in Figs. 4 and 5. Although traditional concepts of ballistics teach that impact kinetic energy is equal to one half the mass of the projectile times velocity squared ($E = 1/2\ MV^2$), the increased energy transmitted from a high-velocity projectile does not necessarily translate to increased wounding capacity. Military-style ammunition is designed to remain intact after striking the intended target, in accordance with the Hague Convention of 1899, and generally is high velocity in nature. Reviewing ballistic studies from the most recent "Emergency War Surgery" manual shows that tissue damage in excess of the diameter of the high-

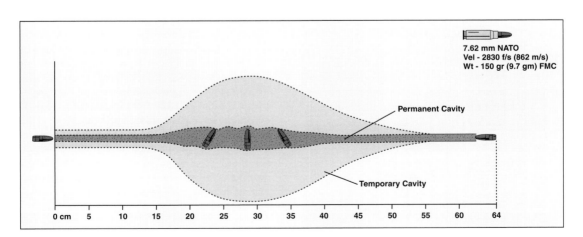

Fig. 4. Wounding characteristics of a 7.62 mm NATO projectile. Note that an increase in permanent cavity size does not occur until 15 cm, and tumbling of the projectile occurs between 20 and 25 cm. *From* United States Government Printing Office. Emergency war surgery. 3$^{rd}$ edition. Washington, DC: United States Government Printing Office; 2004. p. 1.9.

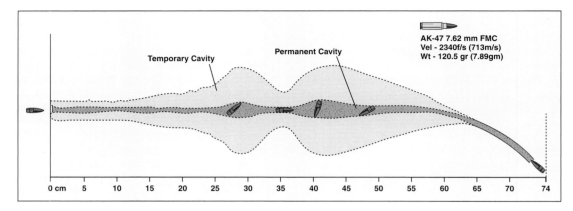

Fig. 5. Wounding characteristics of an AK47 projectile. Note that an increase in permanent cavity size does not occur until 25 cm, and tumbling of the projectile occurs at approximately 35 cm. *From* United States Government Printing Office. Emergency war surgery. 3<sup>rd</sup> edition. Washington, DC: United States Government Printing Office; 2004. p. 1.7.

velocity projectile does not occur until approximately 15 cm into the body of the target when struck with a 7.62-mm NATO round and 25 cm into the body when struck with an AK47 round. The cause for this increase in tissue damage is the backward flip of these projectiles to a reverse trajectory once they strike the body. This change allows for a scenario in which all of the projectile's potential energy may not be transferred into the target, which decreases the wounding potential and tissue damage. Depending on the site of impact, a high-velocity projectile actually could enter and exit the body before breakage or deformation of the projectile and effectively leave minimal tissue injury. Whereas $1/2 MV^2$ relates the potential for tissue injury, the determination of actual injury imparted is related to the construction of the projectile, such as a hollow point that allows expansion versus a bullet that resists deformation, and the projectile's ultimate fate upon striking the target. Fackler [1,2,13] reported extensively that even experienced civilian practitioners who work in urban trauma centers are unable to delineate the injury pattern of low- versus high-velocity projectiles by clinical observation.

## Myth 4: Full metal jacketed bullets always cause greater tissue injuries to a patient

In the late nineteenth century, the velocity of small arm projectiles increased to more than 2400 ft/s (731 m/s), largely because of the development of jacketed bullets in which the soft lead core projectile was covered with a jacket of harder metal [2]. British troops fighting in India were using a new high-

velocity rifle but noted that the weapon did not have the expected increase in severity of wounds on enemy combatants. The British troops filed off the tips of the projectiles to allow for mushrooming of the round and increased damage to enemy troops. Most of the rounds were manufactured at the Dum-Dum arsenal located in India, and the altered ammunition became known as "Dum-Dum" rounds [2,14].

The Hague Convention of 1899 outlawed the use of these modified rounds, and the wounding potential of military ballistics was altered. The specifications of the Hague Convention are strict, and new weapon systems are held to these standards. If a projectile displays excessive fragmentation and tissue injury, recommendations are made to decrease the effectiveness and decrease lethality. High-velocity hunting projectiles and other ammunition available in the civilian community do not follow the Hague Convention recommendations and are designed to tear apart upon discharge, much like the Dum-Dum modification, cause tremendous tissue damage, and impart more of the ballistic energy to the victim. True full metal jacketed military projectiles (Fig. 6) are designed to wound, not kill. Although this idea may seem contradictory to the basic philosophy of warfare, the scenario is different in a military setting than those encountered when hunting or in civilian shootings. Military members are required to transport their own ammunition into battle, and smaller, compact projectiles are easier for soldiers to carry, which increases the number of bullets available for combat. Their ammunition must be able to penetrate armor plating, flak jackets, or other impediments and preferably be fired from a distance that allows the soldiers to remain in relative safety. Barring modi-

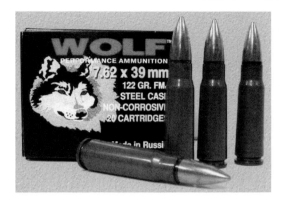

Fig. 6. Military-style full metal jacket ammunition. Note that the hard copper covering completely encases the soft lead projectile. Advertisements for this type of ammunition usually hold the disclaimer of not being recommended for hunting.

fications to the projectile design, they are prone to remain intact after firing, which makes them more likely to pass through the victim. Wounded soldiers have a tremendous psychological impact on unit morale. They also require a significant expenditure of money and additional personnel to assist in transport to medical treatment and provide safety and security during the transfer. If soldiers feel that they or their comrades will not be cared for if injured, combat effectiveness deteriorates rapidly. The ultimate goal in hunting is to inflict tremendous physical damage and kill a target rapidly and in as humane a way as possible. This goal is accomplished principally by the use of ammunition that allows deformation of the projectile almost immediately after release from the barrel of the weapon, such as hollow-point or soft-point ammunition, and does not have the entire projectile covered by the hard casing. Unfortunately, this is the same style ammunition used in many civilian shootings.

## Myth 5: Full metal jacketed ammunition does not fragment, except in unusual situations

This myth is an interesting corollary to the previous myth, which is likely the result of medical providers having a basic understanding of the principle behind full metal jacketed ammunition but not fully comprehending the differences in the projectiles expelled from the shell casing. This is best evaluated by reviewing the line from the previous section: "barring modifications to the projectile design." The United States military committed years

of research and development dollars and expertise to design a ballistic projectile that would inflict the maximum damage to enemy combatants but still be within the accords of the Hague Convention regarding military ballistics. The outcome of this research was the M-193 bullet of the M16A1 rifle, the mainstay of the foot soldier for the United States [15]. This projectile is designed to fragment consistently at the level of the cannulure (Fig. 7), a crimping in the projectile casing behind the tip of the bullet, at approximately 12 cm of tissue in soft tissue only [15]. Any alteration in the projectile design, such as a hollow-tip or soft-point bullet (Fig. 8), has a tremendous increase in the wounding potential of the weapon (Fig. 9) but cannot be considered a true "full metal jacket" round. If the projectile strikes any hard object, such as a building or bone, one would expect to see fragmentation of the bullet. To appreciate better the differences in full metal jacketed projectile injury potential, compare the wound profiles of the M16 (Fig. 10) with the NATO 7.62-mm round (see Fig. 4) and the AK47 (see Fig. 5).

## Myth 6: High-velocity projectile wounds require wide excision for adequate treatment

Rybeck [18] initially reported in 1974 that temporary tissue stretch from high-velocity projectile strikes caused tissue injury up to 30 times the bullet diameter. This information was accepted erroneously and reported in the 1975 edition of the "NATO War Emergency Surgery" manual, which expanded the dimensions to 30 to 40 times the diameter of the projectile and led to a generation of military and civilian surgeons being exposed to this doctrine in their training [28]. Lindsey [29] commented on this phenomenon, which was described as the "idolatry of velocity," and was one of the first to report in the literature regarding the fallacy of this thinking. Although corrected in the 1988 edition of the "War Emergency Surgery" manual, wide acceptance of this practice still exists [30]. If a surgeon applies this concept to the standard 7.62-mm NATO projectile, a patient would experience almost 225 to 300 mm (approximately 10 in) of tissue resection for any

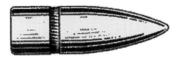

Fig. 7. Cannulure.

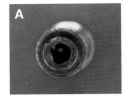
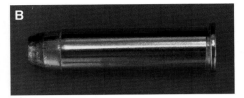

Fig. 8. Hollow-point bullet. (*A*) A hollow cylinder is manufactured into the tip, which allows for expansion of the projectile and increased soft tissue injury. (*B*) Note that the hard copper casing does not cover the entire soft lead projectile.

injury sustained by a high-velocity projectile. Based on this principle, essentially any extremity wound would force the treating surgeon to sacrifice the limb. This concept of automatic amputation is not advocated in any reputable medical literature, nor is it the current standard of care for ballistic injuries to the extremities. Many gunshot wounds in civilian trauma and military settings are from an unknown assailant using an unidentified weapon. Confusion in battle or a crime scene setting does not necessarily allow for proper identification of the weapon used in the assault. No doubt many individuals with high-velocity projectile injuries are not identified as high-velocity projectile victims and are successfully treated conservatively with judicious use of débridement, leaving the wound open, antibiotic therapy, and observation. Although the intent is not to imply that high-velocity wounds never need excision of injured or necrotic tissue, this decision should be made

based on objective clinical findings and not made automatically because a patient was shot by a high-velocity projectile.

**Myth 7: High-velocity projectiles yaw in flight and create irregular wounds**

"Yaw" describes the phenomenon by which a projectile continues on the original path but no longer points directly at the target. This is evidenced by reviewing the ballistic patterns of the NATO 7.62-mm and AK47 projectiles (see Figs. 4 and 5), which show the position of the projectile flipping backward but continuing on the initial path of entry. This change in position is not observed until after contact with the target has occurred, however. Military high-velocity projectiles are designed to travel straight without deflection, and unless the projectile

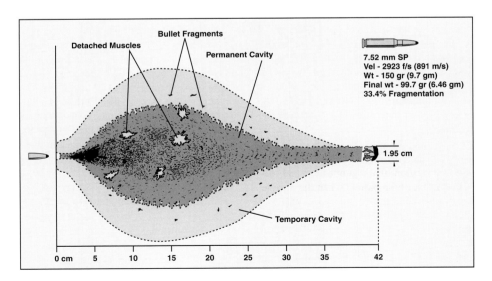

Fig. 9. Wound profile caused by a NATO 7.62-mm cartridge loaded with a soft-point hunting projectile. Note the increased tissue damage that occurs almost immediately upon entering the tissue as the bullet expands and deforms. Compare this profile with the conventional full metal jacketed projectile portrayed in Fig. 4. *From* United States Government Printing Office. Emergency war surgery. 3rd edition. Washington, DC: United States Government Printing Office; 2004.

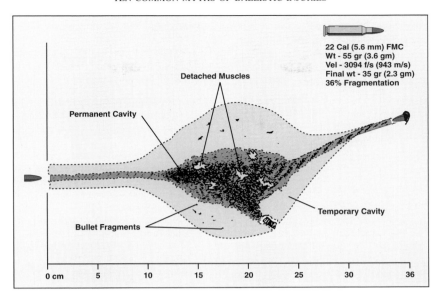

Fig. 10. Wound profile of the M16. Note fragmentation of the projectile at approximately 12 cm into the tissue and the tissue damage comparable to the 7.62 NATO round equipped with a soft-point hunting projectile. *From* United States Government Printing Office. Emergency war surgery. 3rd edition. Washington, DC: United States Government Printing Office; 2004. p. 1.8.

strikes an intermediate target in flight, the amount of yaw is clinically insignificant [15]. The creation of irregular wounding patterns is caused by the composition and design of the projectile itself instead of the yaw or any gyrations in flight before impacting tissue.

## Myth 8: Weapons fired from closer range cause significantly more tissue injury than those fired from a distance

This myth is a potentially confusing statement that is true only in two scenarios: (1) when the weapon is actually touching the patient at discharge and (2) when patients are victims of shotgun blasts. Powder gases are expelled from the muzzle of the weapon after combustion of the gunpowder and follow the projectile out of the barrel. When the muzzle of the weapon is in contact with the target, this can be an additional source of tissue displacement, injury, and thermal burning [1]. Shotgun pellet injuries essentially depend completely on the distance the weapon is from the target at the time of discharge. Sherman and Parrish [31] devised a classification system to describe shotgun wounds in relation to the distance from the target. Type I injury occurs from a distance longer than 7 yards; type II injury is sustained when the discharge is within 3 to 7 yards;

type III injury is within 3 yards. Type III injuries usually sustain dramatic soft and hard tissue injuries and avulsion of tissue, whereas type I injuries may be minimal.

Because victims often have difficulty in determining how far away the shotgun was at the time of discharge, Glezer and colleagues [32] revised this classification system and directed their attention to the size of the pellet scatter. Type I injuries occur when pellet scatter is within an area of 25 cm$^2$; type II injuries are within 10 cm$^2$ to 25 cm$^2$; type III injuries have pellet scatter less than 10 cm$^2$. Although the Glezer classification originally was developed for abdominal injuries, the information is transferable to other areas of the body, and determinations of tissue injury can be correlated directly to the size of the pellet scatter; clinical significance in the head and neck region may be limited. Intuitively, the closer the shotgun is to the patient, the more dramatic the hard and soft tissue damage is. For rifles and handguns, the clinical difference in whether the weapon was 10 feet, 100 feet, or 1000 feet away from the patient otherwise has no bearing on treatment. The range of a .22 caliber handgun is approximately 1 mile, whereas the range of a rifle can be as long as 3 to 4 miles [33]. Although one could argue that at the outer limit of a projectile range it is less likely to penetrate a target, rarely does a shooting occur outside the effective range of a weapon. As a clinician, the determination of distance cannot be calculated in most cases, and even if known, the distance does not alter the basic principles of treatment. A full metal jacket rifle wound from 25 feet is the same as a wound from a rifle at 1000 feet. Tissue injury is caused by the characteristics of projectile shape, design, and composition in relation to velocity at impact, not an absolute correlation to the distance the projectile traveled.

## Myth 9: Exit wounds are always larger than entrance wounds

Simply stated, this statement is untrue and has no bearing on surgical care [15]. Depending on the site of projectile impact and type of bullet used, the entrance and exit wounds likely will be small with minimal tissue disruption.

## Myth 10: Weapon projectiles are considered sterile because of superheating in the chamber

Originally proved false by LaGarde in 1892, confusion still exists as to the possibility of bullets being sterilized after firing because of the high temperatures in the barrel [2,34]. Studies have shown that as bullets penetrate the skin and clothing, they are inoculated with bacteria that are present, and these bacteria are transported into the tissues of the victim [2,7,14,35]. Bullet wounds should be considered contaminated, and appropriate surgical treatment, including saline washouts and antibiotic therapy, are to be initiated.

## Summary

The science of ballistics can be confusing. Specific treatment dogmas regarding ballistic injuries should be examined to ensure that they are supported by scientific data. If determined to be unfounded, these dogmas should be discontinued from the teaching centers and eliminated from clinical practice. Tissue injury by ballistic projectiles is caused by the design and composition of a bullet and the velocity it is traveling when it strikes a target. Velocity or projectile shape alone cannot be the basis for any treatment. Each wound must be evaluated individually, with the determination of care decided by fact and clinical assessment, not rigid treatment protocols.

## References

[1] Fackler ML. Civilian gunshot wounds and ballistics: dispelling the myths. Emerg Med Clin North Am 1998; 16:17–28.

[2] Fackler ML. Gunshot wound review. Ann Emerg Med 1996;28:194–203.

[3] Fackler ML. The wound and the human body: damage pattern correlation. Wound Ballistics Review 1994; 1:12–9.

[4] Fackler ML, Breteau JPL, Sendowski ICP, et al. Perforating wounds of the abdomen by the modern assault rifle. Chungking, China; Proceedings of the Sixth International Wound Ballistics Symposium. J Trauma 1990;6(Suppl):192–9.

[5] Fackler ML. Wounding patterns of military rifle bullets. International Defense Review 1989;1:59.

[6] Fackler ML. War wound treatments. Br J Surg 1989; 76:1217.

[7] Fackler ML, Breteau JP, Courbil LJ, et al. Open wound drainage versus wound excision in treating the modern assault rifle wound. Surgery 1989; 105:576.

[8] Fackler ML, Bellamy RF, Malinowski JA. The wound profile: illustration of the missile-tissue interaction. J Trauma 1988;28:S21.

[9] Fackler ML. Handgun bullet performance. International Defense Review 1988;21:555.

[10] Fackler ML. Wound ballistics: a review of common misconceptions. JAMA 1988;259:2730–6.

[11] Fackler ML. Physics of missile injuries. In: McSwain NE , Kestein MD, editors. Evaluation and management of trauma. Norwalk (CT): Appleton-Century-Crofts; 1987. p. 25–41.

[12] Fackler ML. Ballistic injury. Ann Emerg Med 1986; 15:1451.

[13] Fackler ML, Malinkowski JA. The wound profile: a visual method for quantifying gunshot wound components. J Trauma 1985;25:522–9.

[14] Santucci RA, Chang YJ. Ballistics for physicians: myths about wound ballistics and gunshot injuries. J Urol 2004;171(4):1408–14.

[15] United States Government Printing Office. Emergency war surgery. Third United States Revision. Washington, DC: United States Government Printing Office; 2004.

[16] Di Maio VJM. Gunshot wounds: practical aspects of firearms, ballistics, and forensic techniques. 2nd edition. Washington, DC: CRC Press; 1999. p. 16–7.

[17] Rich NM, Johnson EV, Dimond Jr FC. Wounding power of missiles used in the Republic of Vietnam. JAMA 1967;199:157–61.

[18] Rybeck B. Missile wounding and hemodynamic effects of energy absorption. Acta Chir Scand 1974; 450(Suppl):5–32.

[19] Bartlett CS. Clinical update: gunshot wound ballistics. Clin Orthop 2003;408:28.

[20] Harvey EN, Korr IM, Oster G, et al. Secondary damage in wounding due to pressure changes accom-

panying the passage of high velocity missiles. Surgery 1947;21:218–39.

[21] Suneson A, Hansson HA, Seeman T. Peripheral high-energy missile hits cause pressure changes and damage to the nervous system: experimental studies on pigs. J Trauma 1987;27:782–9.

[22] Suneson A, Hansson HA, Seeman T. Central and peripheral nervous system damage following high-energy missile wounds in the thigh. J Trauma 1988; 28(Suppl 1):S197–203.

[23] Suneson A, Hansson HA, Lycke E, et al. Pressure wave injuries to rat dorsal root ganglion cells in culture caused by high-energy projectiles. J Trauma 1989;29: 10–8.

[24] Suneson A, Hansson HA, Seeman T. Pressure wave injuries to the nervous system caused by high-energy missile extremity impact. I. Local and distant effects on the peripheral nervous system: a light and electron microscopic study on pigs. J Trauma 1990;30: 281–94.

[25] Ordog GJ, Balasubramanian S, Wasserberger J, et al. Extremity gunshot wounds. I. Identification and treatment of patients at high risk of vascular injury. J Trauma 1994;36:358–68.

[26] Barach E, Tomlanovich M, Nowak R. Ballistics:

a pathophysiologic examination of the wounding mechanisms of firearms. Part I. J Trauma 1986;26:225.

[27] Ziervogel JF. A study of the muscle damage caused by the 7.62 NATO rifle. Acta Chir Scand Suppl 1979; 489:131.

[28] United States Government Printing Office. Emergency war surgery: NATO handbook. Washington, DC: United States Government Printing Office; 1975.

[29] Lindsey D. The idolatry of velocity, or lies, damn lies, and ballistics. J Trauma 1980;20:1068.

[30] United States Government Printing Office. Emergency war surgery. NATO handbook. Second United States Revision. Washington, DC: United States Government Printing Office; 1988.

[31] Sherman RT, Parrish RA. Management of shotgun injuries: a review of 152 cases. J Trauma 1963;3:76.

[32] Glezer JA, Minard G, Croce MA, et al. Shotgun wounds to the abdomen. Am Surg 1993;59:129.

[33] Barrish E. Ballistic and explosive injuries: trauma wounds. Audio Digest Emergency Medicine 1998;15(9).

[34] LaGarde LA. Gunshot injuries. 2nd edition. New York: William Wood & Co.; 1916. p. 132.

[35] Adams DB. Wound ballistics: a review. Mil Med 1982;147:831.

ELSEVIER
SAUNDERS

Oral Maxillofacial Surg Clin N Am 17 (2005) 261 – 266

ORAL AND
MAXILLOFACIAL
SURGERY CLINICS
of North America

# Blood Substitutes: Hemoglobin-Based Oxygen Carriers

Colleen M. Fitzpatrick, MD[a],*, Jeffrey D. Kerby, MD, PhD[b]

[a]Department of Surgery, Wilford Hall Medical Center, 2200 Berquist Drive, Suite 1, Lackland AFB, TX 78236, USA
[b]Department of Surgery, University of Alabama at Birmingham, LHRB 112, 701 South 19th Street, Birmingham,
AL 35294-0007, USA

The development of oxygen-carrying red cell substitutes has been an area of intensive research and development since as early as 1917 [1]. Many modifications to hemoglobin solutions have been made in pursuit of an ideal red cell substitute. Early stroma-free hemoglobin solutions were unsuccessful secondary to problems with renal toxicity [2]. To avoid this complication, various techniques have been used to develop hemoglobin-based oxygen carriers (HBOCs), including the use of recombinant technology, polymerization of modified human hemoglobin, and polymerization of bovine hemoglobin [3]. Currently, the most promising agents are the polymerized HBOC solutions, with some of these products undergoing or having recently completed testing in clinical trials [4–8]. HBOCs do not require cross-matching, have long shelf lives, are efficient oxygen transporters, and, in many instances, do not require refrigeration [9]. Currently, no HBOC products have been approved for use by the US Food and Drug Administration, although one product, HBOC-201 (Hemopure) (Biopure Corp., Cambridge, Massachusetts), has been approved for use in South Africa.

HBOCs have significant potential for use in military and civilian settings. Soldiers injured in combat frequently require prompt medical attention; however, tactical combat environments make provision of care a challenge. Injuries are typically sustained in austere settings, often with ongoing hostilities and limited medical resources. The time of evacuation to higher echelons of care varies because of geography and the nature of combat operations. Historically, up to 90% of deaths caused by injuries sustained during combat occur before a soldier reaches a medical treatment facility [10,11]. Current combat resuscitation guidelines call for the use of colloid solutions administered in limited volumes. The US Department of Defense Committee on Tactical Combat Casualty Care has recognized that the ideal fluid for field resuscitation remains elusive [12]. HBOCs may represent a better choice for military field resuscitation fluids.

Many civilian scenarios present challenges similar to military field operations, including large-scale accidents, natural and man-made disasters, and long transport times to trauma centers. HBOCs also represent a safe alternative to blood transfusion when infectious disease transmission is a concern. Whereas the safety of blood banks in the United States continues to improve with regard to hepatitis and HIV, the rate of disease transmission through blood transfusion remains high in many countries throughout the world. The risk of emergence of new pathogens transmitted via blood is unknown, and HBOCs may provide a safer option. Additional civilian applications of HBOCs may include perioperative hemodilution, increased effectiveness of cancer therapies, treatment of sepsis-induced hypotension, preservation of donor organs, treatment of hemolytic anemia, and providing an alternative to blood transfusion for patients who refuse donor blood [13].

Several preclinical studies have demonstrated the safety and efficacy of HBOCs for use in resuscitation after traumatic injury. McNeil and colleagues [14]

* Corresponding author.
 E-mail address: colleen.fitzpatrick@LACKLAND.AF.MIL (C.M. Fitzpatrick).

1042-3699/05/$ – see front matter. Published by Elsevier Inc.
doi:10.1016/j.coms.2005.04.002

investigated the use of HBOC-201 using a swine model of controlled hemorrhage. The study found that when compared with standard resuscitation regimens, hypotensive resuscitation with HBOC-201 provided sufficient tissue perfusion and oxygen delivery to reverse anaerobic metabolism. Using a similar model, York and colleagues [15] found HBOC-201 to be equally safe when compared with standard resuscitation fluids after a 4-hour hypotensive resuscitation with 3-day survival. The work was subsequently expanded to an 8-hour low-volume resuscitation followed by a 5-day survival period. No differences in markers of resuscitation or long-term organ function were identified when HBOC-201 was compared with the current combat regimen that uses a colloid solution. There also was a higher rate of survival in the HBOC group, although the study was underpowered for this difference to achieve statistical significance [16].

Knudson and colleagues [17] found that HBOC-201 was more effective than lactated Ringer's solution or hypertonic saline dextran at restoring blood pressure after controlled hemorrhage. Sampson and colleagues [18] showed that hypotensive resuscitation with HBOC-201 did not produce differences in lactate, base excess, or oxygen consumption levels despite persistently decreased cardiac output, mixed venous saturation levels, and urinary output. A significantly smaller volume of HBOC-201 was required to achieve the same resuscitation endpoints when compared with other standard resuscitation fluids. The decreased volume needed may provide a logistical advantage in various resuscitation scenarios, particularly in the military setting, in which supplies may be limited secondary to logistical constraints.

HBOC-201 infusion causes an increase in vascular resistance that likely accounts for the decreased volume required. The increased resistance has been widely attributed to nitric oxide binding, and it has been noted that the degree of nitric oxide binding may vary with different hemoglobin solutions [19]. However, a study designed to specifically evaluate the effect of HBOC-201 nitric oxide scavenging on vascular reactivity found that the vasoconstrictive effect of HBOC-201 cannot be attributed to nitric oxide scavenging alone [20]. Alternative mechanisms for increased vascular resistance have been proposed, including enhanced endothelin production [21,22], increased oxygen delivery [23], and enhancement of the pressor effects of catecholamines [24]. The vasoactive properties of HBOC-201 do not seem to affect delivery of oxygen to the brain and other vital organs [25]. Researchers also have noted that although HBOCs may cause increased vascular re-

sistance, certain clinical situations exist, such as hypotension in a postoperative cardiac patient, in which the vasoconstrictive effect of HBOCs may be advantageous [26].

In a study that compared PolyHeme (Northfield Laboratories, Evanston, Illinois) to red cells as the initial resuscitation fluid after acute blood loss from surgery or trauma, the vascular response of a subset of patients who required pulmonary artery catheterization was evaluated. No differences were noted between groups (PolyHeme versus packed red cells) for mean arterial pressure, pulmonary artery pressure, cardiac index, or systemic or pulmonary vascular resistance. The authors attributed this to the large size of the polymerized molecule, which prevented the molecule from diffusing out of the intravascular space and interfering with the effect of nitric oxide at the level of the vascular smooth muscle. They also acknowledged that other pathways, such as endothelin or prostacyclin, may be responsible for the effects observed [27].

The vasoactivity and other properties of HBOCs may be helpful in combating the derangements of septic shock. For example, sepsis causes an increase in nitric oxide levels and vasodilation. Presumed nitric oxide scavenging (or alternative pathways) and the resultant increased vascular tone of different HBOC solutions may effectively treat these vasomotor manifestations of sepsis. By definition shock is the inability to provide sufficient oxygen delivery. Because of either modification of the human hemoglobin molecule or use of bovine hemoglobin (higher $P_{50}$ on the oxygen dissociation curve), several of the HBOCs are more efficient at oxygen delivery, and may therefore be useful in the treatment of shock. HBOCs also have a high colloid osmotic pressure which may help to combat the third spacing of fluids during a septic event [28]. Recent animal studies support the use of HBOCs in treating sepsis [29–32]; however, considerable research still must be conducted in this area.

In addition to controlled hemorrhage models, studies of HBOCs in animal models that simulate uncontrolled hemorrhage also have been performed. When compared with lactated Ringer's solution, HBOC-201 vastly improved early survival and stabilized hemodynamic and metabolic parameters in an exsanguinating liver injury model that mimicked the prehospital setting, in which red blood cells are unavailable [33]. HBOC-201 also was found to be superior to no resuscitation or colloid solution resuscitation in this same model, with only HBOC-201 resuscitated animals surviving the injury [34]. In an uncontrolled perioperative hemorrhage model, a recombinant HBOC was found to be superior to lactated Ringer's solution and diaspirin cross-linked hemoglobin (earlier generation HBOC) and was as effective as heterologous blood for maintaining cardiac output and oxygen delivery [35].

Human trials evaluating the use of HBOCs also have been performed. Gould and colleagues [36] reported on the use of polymerized human hemoglobin in the setting of trauma and urgent surgery. They concluded that PolyHeme safely maintained total hemoglobin levels, decreased the need for allogeneic blood transfusions, and effectively loaded and unloaded oxygen. This group reported the first randomized trial that compared polymerized human hemoglobin to red cell transfusion. In that study, patients received either PolyHeme or red cells as the initial resuscitation fluid after acute blood loss from trauma or surgery. Again, PolyHeme safely maintained total hemoglobin levels and decreased the amount of total red cell transfusions needed [5]. A subsequent evaluation of the use of PolyHeme was performed in the setting of massively bleeding patients, in whom larger volumes of the product were infused. The study found that in the absence of red cell transfusion, the infusion of PolyHeme increased survival [6]. PolyHeme currently is being evaluated for use in the prehospital trauma setting, a situation in which blood is not currently available. Another study to evaluate HBOC-201 in the prehospital trauma setting will begin shortly.

With HBOCs being used in acute resuscitation after hemorrhage, the immunomodulatory effect of HBOCs has been of particular interest. The increasing understanding of the role of inflammatory mediators in the development of multisystemic organ failure and the possibility of altering these mediators have spurred much of the interest in this particular area of HBOC research. An in vitro study of oxidative burst and CD11b expression in whole blood exposed to increasing concentration of resuscitation fluids found increased CD11b expression in samples exposed to the maximum concentration of HBOC-201 [37]. Toussaint and colleagues [38] found that whole blood mixed with various hemoglobin solutions (Hb Dex-BTC, $\alpha\alpha$-Hb, and o-raffinose-poly-Hb) did not show evidence of neutrophil activation or changes in expression of the adherence receptors CD62L, CD11b, or CD18. In vivo studies that compared trauma patients transfused with either packed red cells or PolyHeme found that when compared with PolyHeme, red cells caused increased priming of neutrophils in the early postinjury period and increased levels of interleukin-8, interleukin-6, and interleukin-10. These differences may have significant implications in the development of multiple organ failure after injury [39,40].

There does not seem to be a clinically significant immune response to the infusion of HBOCs. In the case of human hemoglobin preparations, there are no cell surface antigens to incite a response. Likewise, the bovine preparations have no surface antigens and the amino acid sequences of the hemoglobin molecules (bovine and human) are sufficiently homologous that there does not seem to be a significant immune response. In a human preoperative hemodilution study, there was no IgE and no sustained IgG response to infusion of HBOC-201 [41]. Hamilton and colleagues [42] investigated the impact on the immune response of repeated doses of a veterinary HBOC preparation in a canine model. Elevated IgG levels were detectable after multiple infusions; however, the levels did not seem to interfere with oxygen binding. No differences were noted between control and HBOC animals for the deposition of IgG, IgA, IgM, and C3 in kidney and liver samples, which indicated no increased risk of antibody-dependent complement-mediated organ damage with the repeated infusions of the HBOC.

HBOCs also have been evaluated for use in the elective surgical setting. One particular application is preoperative hemodilution. Standl and colleagues [41] evaluated the use of HBOC-201 for hemodilution in patients undergoing liver resection, a group of patients in whom allogeneic blood transfusion has been shown to increase postoperative rates of infection and decrease disease-free survival. In this particular study, patients underwent preoperative autologous blood donation with subsequent administration of lactated Ringer's solution and either colloid solution or HBOC-201. The patients who received HBOC-201 demonstrated a higher degree of leukocytosis and reticulocytosis in the early postoperative period. No other significant differences were noted between groups, including transfusion of allogeneic blood or duration of hospital stay. Although there was no clear advantage to the use of HBOC-201 versus colloid, the administration of HBOC-201 was well tolerated and safe. Kasper and colleagues [43] reported on the use of HBOC-201 in preoperative hemodilution for elective abdominal aortic surgery. HBOC-201 caused increased mean arterial pressure and systemic vascular resistance over baseline, whereas cardiac index, oxygen delivery, and oxygen consumption decreased. The authors concluded that HBOC-201 impaired oxygen delivery secondary to decreased cardiac output. Hill and colleagues [44] reported on the use of a different product, Hemolink (Hemosol, Inc., Toronto, Ontario,

Canada), for patients undergoing coronary artery bypass grafting. In that study, Hemolink caused an increase in mean arterial pressure; however, it reduced the volume of allogeneic blood transfused and did not cause any other significant side effects.

Standl and colleagues [45] performed a canine study to evaluate HBOC-201 administration after hemodilution. In the study, dogs were diluted to a hematocrit of 10% followed by administration of either HBOC-201 or packed red cells. HBOC-201 provided faster and higher increases in muscle tissue oxygen tension while maintaining enhanced oxygen extraction. Additional animal hemodilution studies show promising results [46–48], although the exact role of HBOCs in preoperative hemodilution remains to be clarified fully.

HBOCs have been evaluated in the setting of elective surgery for the treatment of intraoperative blood loss. A multicenter study that evaluated the use of HBOC-201 compared with lactated Ringer's solution for intraoperative blood loss found that HBOC-201 was generally well tolerated by patients. Whereas HBOC-201 did not decrease the need for overall blood transfusions, there were no significant adverse events [49]. La Muraglia and colleagues [50] demonstrated a decreased need for blood transfusion when higher doses of HBOC-201 were given to patients who underwent infrarenal aortic reconstruction. HBOC-201 administered in the postoperative period also was found to reduce the need for allogeneic transfusion in up to one third of patients undergoing cardiac surgery [26].

Several additional uses of HBOCs have been reported. HBOCs have been used to treat critically anemic patients who otherwise would have refused blood transfusion secondary to religious beliefs. The most notable faith system that prevents acceptance of allogeneic blood transfusions is that of Jehovah's Witnesses. However, cell-free hemoglobin substitutes are acceptable to this group. Several successful cases that involved use of HBOCs (polymerized bovine and polymerized human hemoglobin) to treat acutely anemic patients have been reported [51–55]. The successful treatment of a Jehovah's Witness patient with acute chest syndrome (a complication of sickle cell disease) has also been reported [56].

Extracorporeal membrane oxygenation is another field in which HBOCs may prove useful. In a healthy porcine model, York and colleagues [57] demonstrated the safety of priming the extracorporeal membrane oxygenation circuit with HBOC-201. There was a decreased need for postpriming volume requirement. The same group conducted a similar experiment using an acute respiratory distress syndrome

model. HBOC-201 again proved to be an effective alternative for pump priming. The authors also cited the advantages of rapid availability and diminished donor cell exposure for a patient on extracorporeal membrane oxygenation [58].

Plastic surgery is yet another area that may benefit from the use of HBOCs. In an animal study of fasciocutaneous flap necrosis, animals were randomized to no treatment, hemodilution with HBOC-201, or hemodilution with lactated Ringer's solution. The animals that received HBOC-201 had significantly decreased flap necrosis when compared with controls and a trend toward decreased necrosis when compared with lactated Ringer's solution. The authors attribute this benefit to the enhanced oxygen transport characteristics of HBOC-201 and its more favorable rheologic properties (decreased viscosity) (Delio Ortegon, MD, unpublished data, 2002).

Blood product substitutes, particularly the HBOCs, represent one of the most exciting fields of research and development in modern medicine. The concept has been several decades in the making, and with products in phase III clinical trials, the use of HBOCs may be close to reality. The potential applications are limitless, with interest expressed from military and civilian sectors.

# References

[1] Amberson WR, Jennings JJ, Rhode CM. Clinical experience with hemoglobin-saline solutions. J Appl Physiol 1949;1:469–89.

[2] Savitsky JP, Doczi J, Black J, et al. A clinical safety trial of stroma-free hemoglobin. Clin Pharmacol Ther 1978;23(1):73–80.

[3] Kim HW, Greenburg AG. Artificial oxygen carriers as red blood cell substitutes: a selected review and current status. Artif Organs 2004;28(9):813–28.

[4] Carmichael FJ. Recent developments in hemoglobin-based oxygen carriers: an update on clinical trials. Transfus Apheresis Sci 2001;24:17–21.

[5] Gould SA, Moore EE, Hoyt DB, et al. The first randomized trial of human polymerized hemoglobin as a blood substitute in acute trauma and emergent surgery. J Am Coll Surg 1998;187:113–20.

[6] Gould SA, Moore EE, Hoyt DB, et al. The life-sustaining capacity of human polymerized hemoglobin when red cells might be unavailable. J Am Coll Surg 2002;195:445–52.

[7] Sprung J, Kindscher JD, Wahr JA, et al. The use of bovine hemoglobin glutamer-250 (Hemopure) in surgical patients: results of a multicenter, randomized, single-blinded trial. Anesth Analg 2002;94:799–808.

[8] Levy JH, Goodnough LT, Greilich PE, et al. Poly-

merized bovine hemoglobin solution as a replacement for allogeneic red blood cell transfusion after cardiac surgery: results of a randomized, double-blind trial. J Thorac Cardiovasc Surg 2002;124:35–42.

[9] Arnoldo BD, Minei JP. Potential of hemoglobin-based oxygen carriers in trauma patients. Curr Opin Crit Care 2001;7:431–6.

[10] Bellamy RF. The causes of death in conventional land warfare: implications for combat casualty care research. Mil Med 1984;149:55–62.

[11] Butler Jr FK, Hagmann JH, Richards DT. Tactical management of urban warfare casualties in special operations. Mil Med 2000;165:1–48.

[12] Prehospital Trauma Life Support Committee of the National Association of Emergency Medical Technicians in cooperation with the Committee on Trauma of the American College of Surgeons. PHTLS: basic and advanced prehospital trauma life support. St. Louis (MO): Mosby; 2003.

[13] Greenburg AG, Kim HW. Civilian uses of hemoglobin-based oxygen carriers. Artif Organs 2004;28(9):795–9.

[14] McNeil JD, Smith DL, Jenkins DH, et al. Hypotensive resuscitation using a polymerized bovine hemoglobin-based oxygen-carrying solution (HBOC-201) leads to reversal of anaerobic metabolism. J Trauma 2001;50:1063–75.

[15] York GB, Eggers JS, Smith DL, et al. Low-volume resuscitation with a polymerized bovine hemoglobin-based oxygen-carrying solution (HBOC-201) provides adequate tissue oxygenation for survival in a porcine model of controlled hemorrhage. J Trauma 2003;55:873–85.

[16] Fitzpatrick CM, Biggs KL, Quance-Fitch FJ, et al. Prolonged low volume resuscitation with HBOC-201 in a large animal survival model of controlled hemorrhage. J Trauma 2004;57(2):448.

[17] Knudson MM, Lee S, Erickson V. Tissue oxygen monitoring during hemorrhagic shock and resuscitation: a comparison of lactated Ringer's solution, hypertonic saline dextran, and HBOC-201. J Trauma 2003;54(2):242–52.

[18] Sampson JB, Davis MR, Mueller DL, et al. A comparison of the hemoglobin-based oxygen carrier HBOC-201 to other low-volume resuscitation fluids in a model of controlled hemorrhagic shock. J Trauma 2003;55:747–54.

[19] Tremper KK. Hemoglobin-based oxygen carriers: problems and promise. J Cardiothorac Vasc Anesth 1997;11:1–2.

[20] Fitzpatrick CM, Savage SA, Kerby JD, et al. Resuscitation with a blood substitute causes vasoconstriction without nitric oxide scavenging in a model of arterial hemorrhage. J Am Coll Surg 2004;199(5):693–701.

[21] Schultz SC, Grady B, Cole F, et al. A role for endothelin and nitric oxide in the pressor response to diaspirin cross-linked hemoglobin. J Lab Clin Med 1993;122:301–8.

[22] Gulati A, Sharma AC, Singh G. Role of endothelin in the cardiovascular effects of diaspirin crosslinked and stroma reduced hemoglobin. Crit Care Med 1996;24:137–47.

[23] Rohlfs RJ, Bruner E, Chiu A, et al. Arterial blood pressure responses to cell-free hemoglobin solutions and the reaction with nitric oxide. J Biol Chem 1998;273:12128–34.

[24] Sharma AC, Gulati A. Yohimbine modulates diaspirin crosslinked hemoglobin-induced systemic hemodynamics and regional circulatory effects. Crit Care Med 1995;23:874–84.

[25] Lee SK, Morabito D, Hemphill C, et al. Small-volume resuscitation with HBOC-201: effects on cardiovascular parameters and brain tissue oxygen tension in an out-of-hospital model of hemorrhage in swine. Acad Emerg Med 2002;9(10):969–76.

[26] Levy JH, Goodnough LT, Greilich PE, et al. Polymerized bovine hemoglobin solution as a replacement for allogeneic red blood cell transfusion after cardiac surgery: results of a randomized, double-blind trial. J Thorac Cardiovasc Surg 2002;124(1):35–42.

[27] Johnson JL, Moore EE, Offner PJ, et al. Resuscitation of the injured patient with polymerized stroma-free hemoglobin does not produce systemic or pulmonary hypertension. Am J Surg 1998;176:612–7.

[28] Creteur J, Vincent JL. Hemoglobin solutions: an "all-in-one" therapeutic strategy in sepsis? Crit Care Med 2000;28(3):894–6.

[29] Kim HW, Messier A, Greenburg AG. Temporal effects of hemoglobin resuscitation on sepsis survival. Artif Cells Blood Substit Immobil Biotechnol 2004;32(3):401–11.

[30] Sielenkamper AW, Eichelbronner O, Martin CM, et al. Diaspirin cross-linked hemoglobin improves mucosal perfusion in the ileum of septic rats. Crit Care Med 2000;28(3):782–7.

[31] Bone HG, Schenarts PJ, Fischer SR, et al. Pyridoxalated hemoglobin polyoxyethylene conjugate reverses hyperdynamic circulation in septic sheep. J Appl Physiol 1998;84(6):1991–9.

[32] Sielenkamper AW, Chin-Yee IH, Martin CM, et al. Diaspirin crosslinked hemoglobin improves systemic oxygen uptake in oxygen supply-dependent septic rats. Am J Respir Crit Care Med 1997;156:1066–72.

[33] Manning JE, Katz LM, Brownstein MR, et al. Bovine hemoglobin-based oxygen carrier (HBOC-201) for resuscitation of uncontrolled exsanguinating liver injury in swine: Carolina Research Group. Shock 2000;13(2):152–9.

[34] Katz LM, Manning JE, McCurdy SL, et al. HBOC-201 improves survival in a swine model of hemorrhagic shock and liver injury. Resuscitation 2002;54:77–8.

[35] Malhotra AK, Kelly ME, Miller PR, et al. Resuscitation with a novel hemoglobin-based oxygen carrier in a swine model of uncontrolled perioperative hemorrhage. J Trauma 2003;54:915–24.

[36] Gould SA, Moore EE, Moore FA, et al. Clinical utility

of human polymerized hemoglobin as a blood substitute after acute trauma and urgent surgery. J Trauma 1997;43(2):325–32.

[37] Ortegon DP, Dixon PS, Crow KK, et al. The effect of the bovine hemoglobin oxygen therapeutic HBOC-201 on human neutrophil activation in vitro. J Trauma 2003;55(4):755–61.

[38] Toussaint M, Latger-Cannard V, Caron A, et al. Effects of three Hb-based oxygen-carrying solution on neutrophil activation in vitro: quantitative measurement of the expression of adherence receptors. Transfusion 2001;41:226–31.

[39] Johnson JL, Moore EE, Offner PJ, et al. Resuscitation with a blood substitute abrogates pathologic postinjury neutrophil cytotoxic function. J Trauma 2001;50(3): 449–56.

[40] Johnson JL, Moore EE, Gonzalez RJ, et al. Alteration of the postinjury hyperinflammatory response by means of resuscitation with a red cell substitute. J Trauma 2003;54(1):133–40.

[41] Standl T, Burmeister MA, Horn EP, et al. Bovine haemoglobin-based oxygen carrier for patients undergoing haemodilution before liver resection. Br J Anaesth 1998;80:189–94.

[42] Hamilton RG, Kelly N, Gawryl MS, et al. Absence of immunopathology associated with repeated IV administration of bovine Hb-based oxygen carrier in dogs. Transfusion 2001;41(2):219–25.

[43] Kasper SM, Walter M, Grune F, et al. Effects of a hemoglobin-based oxygen carrier (HBOC-201) on hemodynamics and oxygen transport in patients undergoing preoperative hemodilution for elective abdominal aortic surgery. Anesth Analg 1996;83(5):912–27.

[44] Hill SE, Gottschalk LI, Grichnik K. Safety and preliminary efficacy of hemoglobin raffimer for patients undergoing coronary artery bypass surgery. J Cardiothorac Vasc Anesth 2002;16(6):695–702.

[45] Standl T, Freitag M, Burmeister MA, et al. Hemoglobin-based oxygen carrier HBOC-201 provides higher and faster increase in oxygen tension in skeletal muscle of anemic dogs than do stored red blood cells. J Vasc Surg 2003;37(4):859–65.

[46] Hare GM, Hum KM, Kim SY, et al. Increased cerebral tissue oxygen tension after extensive hemodilution with a hemoglobin-based oxygen carrier. Anesth Analg 2004;99(2):528–35.

[47] Caron A, Mayer JC, Menu P, et al. Measurement of blood volume after haemodilution with haemoglobin-based oxygen carriers by a radiolabelled-albumin method. Transfus Med 2001;11(6):433–42.

[48] Kingma Jr JG, Sandhu R, Hamelin ND, et al. The effects of hemodilution with Hemolink upon hemodynamics and blood flow distribution in anesthetized dogs. Artif Cells Blood Substit Immobil Biotechnol 2001;29(6):465–81.

[49] Sprung J, Kindscher JD, Wahr JA, et al. The use of bovine hemoglobin glutamer-250 (Hemopure) in surgical patients: results of a multicenter, randomized, single-blinded trial. Anesth Analg 2002;94(4): 799–808.

[50] La Muraglia GM, O'Hara PJ, Baker WH, et al. The reduction of allogeneic transfusion requirement in aortic surgery with a hemoglobin-based solution. J Vasc Surg 2000;31(2):299–308.

[51] Anton N, Hitzler JK, Kavanagh BP. Treatment of life-threatening post-haemorrhagic anaemia with cell-free haemoglobin solution in an adolescent Jehovah's Witness. Br J Haematol 2002;118:1183–6.

[52] Cothren C, Moore EE, Offner PJ, et al. Blood substitute and erythropoietin therapy in a severely injured Jehovah's Witness. N Engl J Med 2002;346(14): 1097–8.

[53] Cothren CC, Moore EE, Long JS, et al. Large volume polymerized haemoglobin solution in a Jehovah's Witness following abruptio placentae. Transfus Med 2004;14:241–6.

[54] Allison G, Feeney C. Successful use of a polymerized hemoglobin blood substitute in a critically anemic Jehovah's Witness. South Med J 2004;97(12):1257–8.

[55] Gannon CJ, Napolitano LM. Severe anemia after gastrointestinal hemorrhage in a Jehovah's Witness: new treatment strategies. Crit Care Med 2002;30(8): 1893–5.

[56] Lanzkron S, Moliterno AR, Norris EJ, et al. Polymerized human Hb use in acute chest syndrome: a case report. Transfusion 2002;42(11):1422–7.

[57] York GB, DiGeronimo RJ, Wilson BJ, et al. Extracorporeal membrane oxygenation in piglets using a polymerized bovine hemoglobin-based oxygen-carrying solution (HBOC-201). J Pediatr Surg 2002;37(10): 1387–92.

[58] Henderson CL, Anderson CM, Sorrells DL, et al. The use of a hemoglobin-based oxygen-carrying solution (HBOC-201) for extracorporeal membrane oxygenation in a porcine model with acute respiratory distress syndrome. Pediatr Crit Care Med 2004;5(4):384–90.

ORAL AND
MAXILLOFACIAL
SURGERY CLINICS
of North America

Oral Maxillofacial Surg Clin N Am 17 (2005) 267 – 272

# Acute Management of Facial Burns

## Shan K. Bagby, DMD

*Department of Oral and Maxillofacial Surgery, Brooke Army Medical Center, 3581 Roger Brooke Drive,
Fort Sam Houston, TX 78234, USA*

Few areas of maxillofacial trauma care are more challenging than the acute management of burn injuries. Facial burns vary from those with relatively minor damage to severe and debilitating injuries. A facial burn can be caused by anything that potentially may burn other body areas, and it rarely occurs in isolation. Facial burns typically cross multiple facial aesthetic subunits and involve varying depths. Such injuries often affect hard and soft tissues and the specialized organs of the eye and respiratory tract, which greatly complicates the diagnosis and initial management picture [1–14].

The mortality associated with delayed recognition or underestimation of the severity of a burn at initial presentation is fairly high. It is imperative that first-contact providers possess the necessary knowledge and skills to assess quickly any patients who have burn injuries. Timely and effective emergency care minimizes morbidity and mortality, facilitates secondary reconstruction, and hastens recovery.

## Soft tissue injury

Skin generally serves as the body's first line of defense against ultraviolet radiation, temperature extremes, toxins, and bacteria. Other significant functions include sensory perception, immunologic surveillance, thermoregulation, and control of insensible fluid loss. The skin consists of three principal layers: the epidermis, the dermis, and an underlying fatty subcutaneous layer. The superficial epidermal layer relies on the underlying dermis for its nutrition because it lacks native blood vessels. The primary function of the dermis is to sustain and support the epidermis.

Dermal appendages, including hair follicles and sebaceous glands, are highly concentrated in the face and scalp and are generally located within the deep dermis. After injury to the epidermis, such as partial-thickness burns or traumatic abrasions, dermal appendages act to re-epithelialize and restore the skin surface. Their deep location and density account for the remarkable ability of the skin to heal after most wounds. Skin thickness varies with anatomic location, sex, and age. The thinnest skin on the body is found on the eyelids and postauricular regions, where the skin may be as thin as 0.5 mm.

Burns to the skin can occur above 48°C and are characterized as being first, second, or third degree, depending on the depth of injury. First-degree or superficial burns typically cause minor skin damage that is confined to the epidermis. A mild sunburn is a classic example of a first-degree burn (Fig. 1). Second-degree or partial-thickness burns destroy the epidermis and a portion of the dermis and are usually painful (Fig. 2). In healthy subjects, most second-degree burns re-epithelialize spontaneously if managed appropriately. Third-degree or full-thickness burns destroy the full depth of the epidermal and dermal layers and are insensate because of sensory nerve damage. These full-thickness burns initially appear grayish, white, or translucent and may progress to brown or black in color during eschar formation (Fig. 3). Third-degree burns rarely heal

*E-mail address:* shan.bagby@us.army.mil

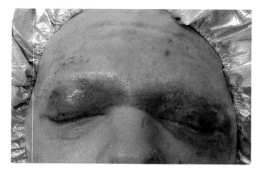

Fig. 1. First- and second-degree burns.

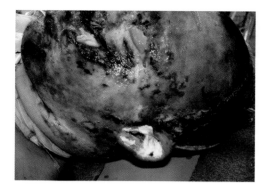

Fig. 3. Third-degree burns.

spontaneously unless they are small, and they may result in disfiguring scarring and contraction.

## Pathophysiology of inhalation injuries

Inhalation injuries are a common occurrence in severe facial burns. Inhalation injury is defined as insult to any portion of the respiratory system as the result of oxygen deprivation or aspiration of the toxic products of incomplete combustion. Three separate components must be considered: asphyxiation with impaired tissue oxygenation, thermal insult to the upper airway, and smoke injury, usually to the lower airway. Early recognition of inhalation injury is crucial. Facial burn victims with inhalation injury initially may present without respiratory dysfunction and may not receive supportive pulmonary therapy in time to prevent morbidity and death. The mortality rate among burned patients with concomitant inhalation injury is double that of patients with cutaneous facial burns alone.

### Asphyxiation

Asphyxiation is characterized by suffocation caused by oxygen deprivation and is an immediate

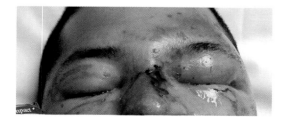

Fig. 2. Second-degree burns.

threat to life. In burn injuries, asphyxiation may occur secondary to decreased oxygen levels, carbon monoxide poisoning, or cyanide poisoning. At the scene of a fire, oxygen levels may be as low as 5% because of the consumption of oxygen in the combustion process, which deprives a victim of oxygen for extended periods.

Carbon monoxide is an odorless, colorless gas produced by incomplete combustion of certain materials. It binds hemoglobin with an affinity 250 times greater than that of oxygen, which inhibits the reversible displacement of oxygen on the hemoglobin molecule. This occurrence produces the characteristic "left shift" in the oxygen-hemoglobin dissociation curve, which causes metabolic acidosis and decreased oxygen carrying capacity. Clinical manifestations of carbon monoxide poisoning include headache, dizziness, abdominal pain, confusion, lethargy, and nausea.

Hydrogen cyanide is produced by burning certain plastics, and it carries a distinctive bitter almond scent. Combined exposure to carbon monoxide and hydrogen cyanide results in a synergistic decrease in tissue oxygen use, the result of which is accelerated lactic acidosis and asphyxia. Carbon monoxide and cyanide poisoning have been implicated in nearly 80% of early fire deaths in enclosed spaces.

In evaluating a patient with suspected asphyxia caused by toxic gas exposure, routine arterial blood gas testing and pulse oximetry may yield falsely normal results. With carbon monoxide poisoning, arterial blood gas $PO_2$ levels may remain normal because the test measures dissolved oxygen, not oxyhemoglobin. Oxyhemoglobin and carboxyhemoglobin absorb light at similar wavelengths and are indistinguishable by most pulse oximetry equipment. The half-life of the carboxyhemoglobin complex is 4 hours in room air but is reduced to 1 hour when high concentrations of oxygen are administered. The elimination half-life of cyanide is relatively short (1.2 hours). One hundred percent oxygen via non-rebreather face mask or endotracheal tube is the treatment of choice in cases of suspected poisoning, followed by arterial blood gas monitoring to evaluate the progress of metabolic acidosis resolution.

*Thermal injury*

Thermal injury to the airway occurs principally because of inhaled heat and manifests clinically as delayed, severe mucosal edema. Most often the injury is restricted to the nasopharynx and oropharynx, with rare involvement of the lower airway, except in cases that involve inhaled steam. Airway burns produce mucosal and submucosal edema, erythema, hemorrhage, and ulceration, which impair ability to clear respiratory secretions, cause upper airway obstruction, and, in severe cases, cause rapid respiratory collapse. First responders should suspect thermal airway injury in cases in which an explosion occurred or a loss of consciousness at the scene is reported. Typical clinical findings include red and dry mucosa accompanied by oral blistering. Inspiratory stridor may be heard on auscultation of the lungs. Direct or fiberoptic laryngoscopy is useful in evaluating the degree of injury, although the presence of carbonaceous debris, edema, or erythema usually confirms the diagnosis.

*Chemical injury*

Visible smoke is comprised of carbon particles that carry more than 300 caustic compounds formed during combustion. The chemical composition varies according to the material burned, oxygen concentration, and heat of combustion. In contrast to thermal insult, chemical injury tends to occur in the lower airway because of particulate deposition in distal airway spaces. Injury to the respiratory epithelium caused by chemical exposure can cause delayed liquefaction necrosis, which manifests initially as simple atelectasis and progresses to airway obstruction. The pathophysiology of pulmonary chemical injury is characterized by three stages. Stage I occurs immediately and results in respiratory epithelial damage. Stage II (inflammatory response) starts 2 hours after initial injury and peaks at 24 to 48 hours. Stage III (bacterial colonization) develops 72 hours after injury and lasts for up to 6 weeks and can lead to severe pulmonary infection.

**Patient evaluation**

*Initial evaluation*

Facial burns rarely occur as an isolated injury. Providers must assess the full extent of injury, including the total body surface area involved and the depth of wounding. When evaluating a patient with severe facial burns, a modified ATLS primary and secondary survey should be performed, with particular emphasis placed on the airway and breathing components. Two key tasks in the initial evaluation of the burned patient are immediate and accurate history taking and serial physical examinations.

The history of injury should be elicited immediately because it may yield clues as to the nature and likely depth of burn and quantify the likelihood of inhalation injury. The mechanism of injury, circumstances, and any prehospital treatment should be ascertained at first contact in case airway swelling and intubation may make it impossible later. A patient's smoking history should be quantified and the effect on serial blood gas values considered. All facial burn victims should receive high-flow humidified oxygen at first contact, and intravenous access should be established, preferably in an unburned distal site. Patients should be reassessed frequently for signs of respiratory distress, and the cervical spine should be protected if a patient presents in an unconscious state.

*Airway management*

Severe facial burns accompanied by inhalation injury may require early intubation. Prophylactic intubation in asymptomatic and closely observed patients is usually unnecessary and is outweighed by the risk of laryngeal or tracheal injury. During the secondary survey, direct inspection of the oropharynx should be performed as a baseline before the onset of edema. If edema is noticeably progressive, then early fiberoptic intubation should be considered. The soft tissues of the face, neck, and chest should be inspected for deep dermal or full-thickness burns that can inhibit adequate ventilation. Blast injuries complicate the clinical picture. Concussive blast forces transmitted in an enclosed space can cause severe pulmonary trauma, including lung contusions and severe alveolar trauma, which lead to adult respiratory distress syndrome in the postinjury period. Blast fragments and debris can cause penetrating injuries and tension pneumothoraces. In all cases, patients should be reassessed frequently for signs of respiratory distress.

If intubation is accomplished, the endotracheal tube can be secured using various acceptable methods, such as direct wiring to the teeth or jaw. Regardless of the method, the tube should be secured in a manner that minimizes soft tissue pressure and leaves room for any delayed facial swelling. Likewise, if a feeding tube is placed, it should be positioned to minimize the risk of alar or columellar necrosis. Emergency cricothyroidotomy should be performed if obstruction is imminent and endotracheal intubation is not possible. Tracheostomy should not be used as the first step in airway management but may be planned if an extended period of intubation is expected. Elective tracheostomy when indicated is typically planned between 3 and 30 days after intubation.

## Ocular injury

The incidence of eye injuries associated with facial burns is as high as 27%. Diagnosis and treatment of thermal ocular injuries are often delayed because associated life-threatening pulmonary injuries require immediate attention and are a distracter. Intense periorbital edema also may make examination difficult, and significant eye injuries may be overlooked initially.

Initial evaluation should include external and funduscopic examination during the secondary survey. Documentation of visual acuity provides a baseline for monitoring any visual changes. Subjective visual complaints, including foreign body sensation, progressive loss of visual acuity, and acute eye pain, are worrisome signs. Globe pressure should be measured or estimated digitally and appropriate measures taken, such as a lateral canthotomy, to relieve globe pressure. The eyelashes are often burned away because of reflexive eyelid closure upon exposure to direct heat. The eyelid itself is thin, transmits heat easily, and readily undergoes contracture and scarring when subject to intense direct heat. This damage can leave the ocular surface exposed and contribute to progressive and irreversible corneal damage if not recognized and treated in time. The exposure can be subtle and is often overlooked when more obvious or life-threatening injuries must be dealt with.

True thermal burns to the globe surface are rare and usually result in severe ocular injury and blindness. Severe midface burns with eyelid sparing suggest open eyes at the time of injury with direct thermal exposure of the globe. Severe conjunctival inflammation and corneal defects may be seen (Fig. 4). Corneal burn defect injuries often require referral

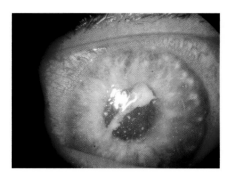

Fig. 4. Ocular burn.

for secondary repair and ocular reconstruction. In most cases, artificial tears, ophthalmic ointments, and patching protect the eyes until consultation with an ophthalmologist can be arranged.

## Initial management

Initial management of severe facial burns should be aimed at preventing airway compromise and death caused by airway edema and pulmonary injury. All patients should receive humidified oxygen by face mask, suctioning to evacuate oral secretions, elevation of the head 30° to promote clearing of secretions, and administration of racemic epinephrine to reduce oropharyngeal edema. Fiberoptic-guided endotracheal intubation is indicated if pending airway compromise is suspected, and should be performed as early as possible. Progressive edema may make delayed intubation difficult or impossible. All patients burned in a fire in which toxin production is suspected should be monitored for 24 hours in an intensive care setting.

The diagnosis of inhalation injury relies heavily on careful review of the history and physical examination. The treatment objectives are to support oxygenation and maintain airway patency. Patients initially may present without respiratory complaints because of the delayed onset of edema. A victim of facial burns in an enclosed environment should be assumed to have severe inhalation injury because less air is present to dilute the inhaled smoke, which results in greater chemical and thermal pulmonary exposure. Ominous clinical signs of inhalation injury in patients with facial burns include carbonaceous sputum, copious mucous production, oronasal soot, wheezing, ronchi hoarseness, singed nasal hair, cough, dyspnea, and oropharyngeal edema. Arterial blood gas levels and oximetry should be augmented with chest radiography as a baseline.

Ocular involvement also should be assessed during the secondary survey to preserve vision. Visual acuity testing provides a baseline for later visual changes and should be repeated periodically. If any ocular injury or lagophthalmos is present, it is important to keep the eyes moisturized with ophthalmic ointment to prevent exposure keratitis. Alternatively, tarsorrhaphy can be considered but is seldom necessary. The affected eye should be patched for protection and to prevent desiccation.

Patients who have been burned experience insensible fluid loss in proportion to injury size, delay in initiation of resuscitation, and the presence of inhalation injury for the first 18 to 24 hours after injury. Fluid resuscitation with Ringer's lactate can begin using one of several formulas. Urine output should be used as a guide to hydration status. A urine output of 0.5 mL/kg/h is an indicator of adequate fluid resuscitation. Patients who are able and willing to take fluid by mouth may be allowed to drink, with additional fluid administered intravenously at a maintenance rate.

Once more life- or sight-threatening concerns are addressed, the facial soft tissues may be gently débrided of blisters and loose tissue in second- and third-degree burns. Initial sharp excision of tissue is not advised because it is often difficult to determine the exact depth of injury, and such action may injure underlying muscles or nerves. Gentle débridement under appropriate anesthesia should be performed, followed by topical ointment application.

The depth of the wound dictates the choice of topical agent. First- and second-degree burns may be treated with sulfadiazine, antibiotic ointment, or petrolatum to help prevent wound desiccation and provide antimicrobial protection. Silver sulfadiazine can be used for third-degree burns and on lesser burns of the ears to prevent chondritis. The face may be washed twice daily with soap and water, after which a topical agent is reapplied. Daily wound care may be continued until definitive burn care is initiated or the patient is transferred to a burn center. With second- and third-degree burns, the application of splints (Hartford or Larson device) to oral commissures and the neck may help prevent contracture development. Appropriate early measures may render subsequent grafting and reconstruction procedures less daunting.

Pain control is an important component of burn management and must not be overlooked. Initially, intravenous morphine or meperidine may be used. If intravenous access is not possible, an oral narcotic medication administered 30 to 60 minutes before a planned dressing change provides adequate pain control. Because most dressings are occlusive, pain control between dressing changes tends to be managed adequately without narcotics. In the initial stage of management, early signs of infection or a wound that appears deeper than appreciated during the initial examination should be investigated.

## Summary

Success in accurately diagnosing and providing first-contact treatment for patients with facial burns relies on accurate history taking, physical examination, and close observation. Providers must understand the early and delayed effects of heat and chemicals on human tissue and the respiratory system. Initial treatment should be aimed at preventing complications and accurately identifying the extent of injury and rapidly administering appropriate therapy. Vigilance is important given the delayed nature of edema caused by burns. Rapid diagnosis and early intervention are key in keeping patients alive and facilitating definitive burn care.

## References

[1] Davis C. Endotracheal tube fixation to the maxilla in patients with facial burns. Plast Reconstr Surg 2004; 113(3):982–4.

[2] Hettiaratchy S. Initial management of a major burn: overview. BMJ 2004;328:1555–7.

[3] Ryan C, Schoenfeld DA. Objective estimates of the probability of death from burn injuries. N Engl J Med 1998;338(6):362–6.

[4] Bouchard C, Morno K, Perkins J. Ocular complications of thermal injury: a 3-year retrospective. J Trauma 2001;50(1):79–82.

[5] Klein J, Moore M, Costa B. Primer on the management of face burns at the University of Washington. J Burn Care Rehabil 2005;26(1):2–6.

[6] Engrav LH, Richey KJ, Walkinshaw MD, et al. Chondritis of the burned ear: a preventable complication. Ann Plast Surg 1989;23:1–2.

[7] McAuliffe PF, Mozingo DW. Inhalation injury and ventilator management. Probl Gen Surg 2003;20: 97–105.

[8] Clark WR. Smoke inhalation: diagnosis and treatment. World J Surg 1992;16:24–9.

[9] Sheridan RL. Airway management and respiratory care of the burn patient. Int Anesthesiol Clin 2000;38: 129–45.

[10] Canio LC, Mozingo DW, Pruitt BA. Strategies for diagnosing and treating asphyxiation and inhalation injuries. J Crit Illn 1997;12:217–29.

[11] Barillo DJ, Goode R, Esch V. Cyanide poisoning in victims of fire: analysis of 364 cases and review of the literature. J Burn Care Rehabil 1994;15:46–57.

[12] Herndon DN, Barrow RE, Linares HA, et al. Inhalation injury in burned patients, effects and treatment. Burns Incl Therm Inj 1988;14:349–56.

[13] Lund T, Goodwin CW, McNanus WF, et al. Upper airway sequelae in burn patients requiring endotracheal intubation or tracheostomy. Ann Surg 1985;201:374–82.

[14] Revis R, Seagel MB. Facial burns. Available at: http://www.emedicine.com/ent/topic627.htm. Accessed November 3, 2004.

ELSEVIER
SAUNDERS

Oral Maxillofacial Surg Clin N Am 17 (2005) 273 – 280

**ORAL AND
MAXILLOFACIAL
SURGERY CLINICS**
of North America

# Distribution of Maxillofacial Injuries in Terrorist Attacks

## Oscar Hasson, DDS

*Department of Oral and Maxillofacial Surgery, Kaplan Medical Center, POB1, Rehovot, Israel*

Terrorist attacks are unfortunately part of the Israeli life, and throughout the years many Israelis have been injured or died because of those acts. In the beginning of the 1970s, bomb attacks occurred either inside of buses or in open-air settings, where a bomb left early in the selected places was the modus operandi of the terrorists. Adler and colleagues [1] reported their experience with terrorist bombings in Israel from 1975 to 1979. In that period, 24 bombs caused 511 casualties. Most of the injuries (39%) were in the lower extremities, because explosives were usually placed in the ground level of buses. The head and neck region was affected in 19.3% of the cases.

An increase in the number and intensity of terrorist attacks occurred during the first Palestinian uprising (Intifada) from 1987 to 1993 and during the second Palestinian uprising (Intifada El-Aqsa) from 2000 until the current time. During the last uprising, a total of 1155 terrorist-related injuries occurred [2]. In each uprising, different weapons were used, which consequently resulted in different types of injuries. During the first Palestinian uprising, blocks and stones, knives, and guns were the preferred weapons used by the terrorists. During the second uprising, a more destructive weapon—suicide bombers—were introduced repeatedly, and they resulted in more devastating and severe injuries.

Because of the high number of terrorist attacks and the need to deal with mass casualties at the same time on short notice, Israeli medical centers—especially trauma one level centers—have developed their own systematic approach that has been used as a model worldwide [2–4].

Israeli oral and maxillofacial surgeons have been involved in the treatment of injured patients in many terrorist attacks and are usually summoned immediately when such attacks take place, because many patients present with involvement of the facial skeleton. Maxillofacial injuries involve the hard and soft tissues, and severity of wounds is related directly to the intensity of the attack and weaponry used. At the end of the 1980s and in the early 1990s, comminutive facial fractures and soft tissue lacerations were common because attackers were throwing stones and blocks and using knives. In the middle of the 1990s, terrorists changed to more sophisticated weapons, such as automatic guns, which caused penetrating and avulsive wounds. The search by terrorists for more aggressive and destructive weapons permitted the "creation" of suicide bombers. Although suicide bombers have been used in the past by others, the Islamic extremist groups popularized them, turning it into a brutal weapon against the Israeli population. Because these attackers detonate their devices in closed- and open-air locations close to their victims, facial burns, soft tissue mutilations, and injuries caused by shrapnel and metal parts attached to the explosive devices are common.

The purpose of this article is to present the different types of maxillofacial injuries sustained by the Israeli population as result of stoning, stabbing, gunshots, and suicide bomb attacks and describe the characteristics and treatment for these unusual types of wounds.

## Stoning injuries

Stoning consists of throwing rocks and blocks toward cars and buses. Civilians and army personnel

*E-mail address:* oshasson@yahoo.com

1042-3699/05/$ – see front matter © 2005 Elsevier Inc. All rights reserved.
doi:10.1016/j.coms.2005.04.001

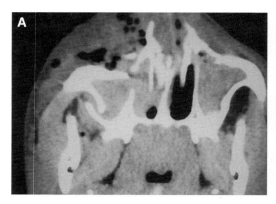 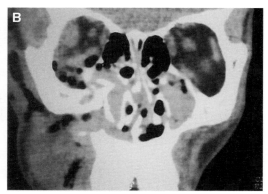

Fig. 1. (*A*) Axial CT scan shows zygomatic bone fracture after a stone throwing. Note the swelling of surrounding soft tissue. (*B*) Coronal CT scan shows comminution pattern of the right zygomatic bone and maxilla.

suffer from these acts. Injured patients suffer from the damage caused by the impact of the stone to body parts, by broken glasses caused by the impact of the stone, or by car accident caused by the impact of the stone on the driver of the vehicle. Experience has shown that damage to hard and soft tissues is more severe in patients hit while traveling inside a vehicle when compared with patients injured as bystanders. Civilians and soldiers are both injured. Heering and colleagues [5] reported on injuries sustained by Israeli soldiers from 1987 to 1989 (the first Palestinian uprising). Of 1267 soldiers injured, 62% were from stones thrown. The skull and neck areas were injured in 195 soldiers and the jaws were injured in 70 soldiers. Frequently, injured patients suffered from

head and facial trauma because those body parts were exposed at the time of the attack.

Maxillofacial injuries that result from stoning are common. In most of the injured persons, the lateral portion of the face is the stone's impact location, which explains the high number of temporal bone fractures and mandibular and zygomatic bone fractures (Fig. 1A, B). CT is the standard radiographic examination performed to evaluate the involvement and damage of the head and facial bones. Bone fractures are mainly comminutive at the hit point area with displacement of fragments (Fig. 2). Some patients also present with more than one fracture site (Fig. 3). Bruises and tissue maceration characterize soft tissue injuries. Cleaning and rinsing of tissues are performed routinely to detect and remove parts of concrete and glasses from inner portions of wounds. In decreasing frequency, other sites injured by stoning and blocks are the zygomatic arch, especially

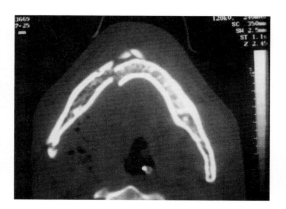

Fig. 2. Axial CT scan shows comminution and severe displacement of a frontal bone fracture after stone throwing.

Fig. 3. Axial CT scan shows comminutive fracture of mandibular symphysis area after stone throwing. Note the presence of a second fracture on the left ascending ramus.

a driver's left side, the midface, alveolar bone, and teeth. All sites present the same pattern of comminutive fractures at hit point.

Nahlieli and colleagues [6] reported their experience in the treatment of 15 patients who suffered from mandibular fractures after stone throwing. Eight patients were driving a vehicle at the time of injury and presented with fracture of the left mandible. They also reported encountering an eggshell-type fracture at the lingual portion of hit area, which did not permit sometimes appropriate reduction of bone fractures by screws and plating.

## Stab wounds

After stoning, stab wounds were the second most common type of injury in the beginning of the 1990s in Israel. In most of the stab wound attacks, terrorists used kitchen or butcher knives as their weapon. Terrorist stabbings are different from civilian acts because terrorists perform their attacks in daylight and in crowded areas [7]. Although most of the victims were men in their twenties or thirties, some of the injured were middle age and older women who were attacked at bus stops while waiting for their bus.

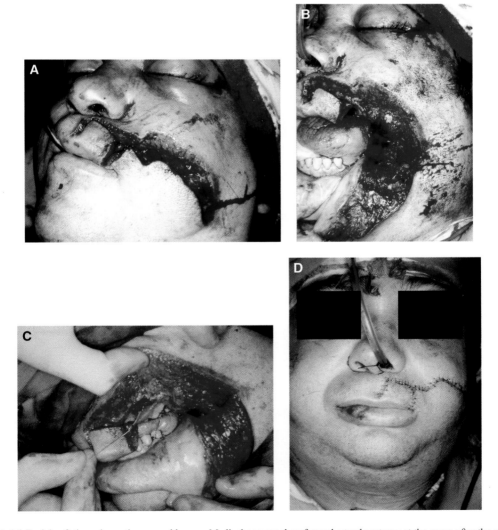

Fig. 4. (*A*) Facial soft tissue laceration caused by axe. Medical personnel performed a tracheostomy at the scene after the attack. (*B*) Opening of the wound for inspection and cleaning disclosed the severity of injuries. (*C*) Checking the integrity of the Stenson's duct. Note the presence of Yvy loops for installation of intermaxillary fixation. (*D*) Immediate postoperative appearance after suturing of facial injuries.

Because of their lack of reflex and impossibility of reaction, they were stabbed repeatedly on different regions of their body. Injuries were severe, and many victims perished at the scene of the attack before receiving medical attention. Hanoch and colleagues [7] reported their experience in the treatment of 154 cases of stab wounds between 1987 and 1994 in Israel. They reported that most of the injuries were located in the right posterior thorax, which demonstrated that the victims were attacked from behind. After the thorax (71 cases), the neck (29 cases) and the head (20 cases) were other anatomic regions commonly involved. There were 39 deaths from the wounds, 31 of which occurred at the scene of the attack. The authors also stressed the need to remove knives from the wounds in a controlled setting to manage possible massive hemorrhage and prevent death after removal of the weapon. They also reported on two patients who were conscious after an attack but died at the scene after the removal of the knife by a bystander in 1 case (stabbed in the left thorax) and by a paramedic in another case (stabbed in the neck).

Stab wounds in the maxillofacial regions usually were the only injury; sometimes they were superficial with an "apparent" clean aspect. In a few cases the face and the head were involved. Some patients presented with concomitant alveolar ridge or mandibular fractures, which disclosed the high intensity of the hit during the attack.

One of the striking cases involved an Israeli citizen who was attacked by terrorists using an axe. He was hit in the face and head and suffered several wounds. From the intensity of the hit, not only was the facial soft tissue badly injured and lacerated (Fig. 4A–D) but also the victim sustained an undisplaced mandibular fracture. He also fractured his hand while defending himself from the attackers. He arrived at the hospital with a tracheostomy that was performed at the scene. Although his wounds were severe, they did not damage important structures, such as facial nerve or Stenson's duct. The patient experienced a full recovery after soft tissue repair and 6 weeks of intermaxillary fixation as treatment for mandibular fracture. Unfortunately, terrorism was present again in this patient's life when, a few years later, a close member of his family was killed in another terrorist attack.

**Gunshot wounds**

Gunshot wounds were sustained by citizens and by army personnel. Citizens were targeted in the

bigger cities of Israel. The usual scenario was that of gunmen appearing suddenly and opening fire in crowded areas, injuring bystanders. In the West Bank and Gaza strip, Israeli citizens and soldiers were targeted, especially while driving on the highways.

Peleg and colleagues [2] reported their study based on the records of the Israeli National Trauma Registry from October 2000 to June 2002. Of 1155 terrorist-related injuries in this period, 36% (410) were the result of gunshot wounds. The chest, spine, and the abdomen were common injured sites. Only 22 (16%) patients suffered injuries to the head.

Maxillofacial injuries from gunshots comprised a small percentage of the anatomic sites of injury when compared with other portions of the body. Most of the injuries were from a high-velocity–type bullet that caused extensive loss of soft and hard tissue when compare with stones and stab wounds (Fig. 5). The usual approach for patients with maxillofacial gunshot wounds injuries consists of re-establishment of the occlusion by intermaxillary fixation with arch bars and minimum tissue débridement. Bone plating usually is not performed, and bone grafting, if needed, is undertaken as a secondary procedure. Patients with extensive loss of soft and hard tissue in the middle third area of the maxillofacial region require reconstruction with a maxillary obturator. Some controversy exists regarding the best approach for gunshot wounds in the maxillofacial region [8]. The chosen surgical approach depends on the type of injury, type of bullet (ie, high or low velocity), amount of tissue lost, and individual expertise and surgical preferences.

Motamedi [9] reported his experience in treating 30 casualties with facial gunshot wounds during the

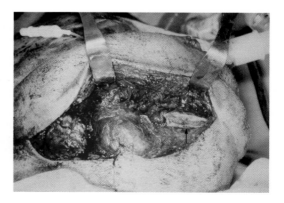

Fig. 5. High-velocity gunshot wound. Note the exit of the projectile, which caused severe damage of soft tissue. The mandible also was injured badly. Only a small portion of the right body region remained (*arrow*).

Iran-Iraq War. The mandible was injured in most cases. Intermaxillary fixation and primary closure of tissues with minimum débridement was performed in most cases. Open reduction using plating or screws was performed in 13% of the cases. Patients with extensive bone loss were treated in a secondary procedure with bone grafting. Sadda [10] reported his experience in the treatment of 300 maxillofacial casualties also during the Iraq-Iran War. Gunshot wounds comprised 19.7% of the cases in which the mandible, especially the body portion, was normally injured. Most fractures were treated by closed reduction.

### Suicide bombings

Suicide bombings became the preferred terrorist weapon and caused severe and brutal injuries to the Israeli population. Crowded sites, such as malls, coffee shops, pedestrian promenades, and buses, were targeted. The result of such acts is mass casualties. Suicide attacks started in the mid-1990s in Israel; however, their intensity and sophistication were felt during the second Palestinian uprising. From November 2000 to May 2003 [4], 71 suicide bombings occurred in Israel. Fifty-two took place in open spaces, 13 detonated inside buses, and 6 occurred in semiconfined spaces (eg, coffees shops and restaurants). During the same period, security forces intercepted and imprisoned 85 other suicide bombers on their way to perform their "mission." The security forces also dealt with more than 40 warnings of potential suicide bombings every day.

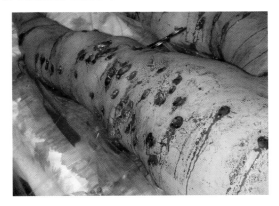

Fig. 7. The left lower limb of a 14-year-old girl who sustained multiple shrapnel injuries. Note the extensive soft tissue damage. (*From* Almogy G, Belzberg H, Mintz Y, et al. Suicide bombing attacks: update and modifications to the protocol. Ann Surg 2004;239(3):302; with permission.)

Suicide bombers commonly use shrapnel, metal bolts, and screws attached to their explosive devices to inflict more severe injuries to superficial and deeper portions of tissues (Figs. 6–8). These metal parts and bolts become airborne and wound not only civilians close to the attacker but also individuals far from the center of the explosion.

Stein and Hirshberg [11], and Kluger [12] identified four phases of medical treatment after a suicide bombing. The first phase is the chaotic phase, which involves the first minutes after the explosion, when no medical forces are present at the scene. Lightly injured civilians leave the area by themselves and arrive at nearby medical centers without help or with help of other civilians. Bystanders help more severely injured persons until the arrival of medical personnel. The second phase is the reorganization

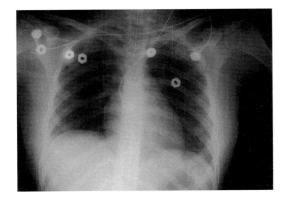

Fig. 6. Chest radiograph of a patient injured after a suicide bombing. In addition to the EKG leads (*solid whites*), note the presence of five metal bolts in this patient's chest. (Courtesy of Z. Gimmon, MD, Jerusalem, Israel.)

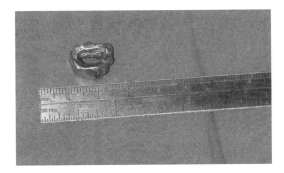

Fig. 8. An "ordinary household" nut removed from the thigh of 19-year-old woman. (*From* Almogy G, Belzberg H, Mintz Y, et al. Suicide bombing attacks: update and modifications to the protocol. Ann Surg 2004;239(3):297; with permission.)

phase, when medical personnel arrive and a medical officer takes charge of the scene. The first goal in the reorganization phase is to identify life-threatening situations and severely injured—but salvageable—patients. These more severe casualties are evacuated before lightly injured patients. This phase lasts approximately 60 minutes. The third phase is the site-clearing phase (100–180 minutes after the blast), when the medical commander re-examines the scene to certify that no one is left behind and that evacuation of the casualties is finished. The fourth phase is the late phase (24–48 hours after the attack), when minimally injured patients who were unaware of their injuries arrive at the hospital (normally with minor bruises) or civilians with emotional stress, sometimes civilians who were not close to the scene, arrive for medical attention.

Because of the high number of suicide bombings and the fact that they happen in different settings, different types of injuries can be identified depending on the characteristics of the explosion area. Explosions that occur in close settings, such as buses, produce more severe injuries and higher percentage of deaths when compared with injuries and deaths from explosions in open-air locations. Explosions in semi-closed areas, such as restaurants, however, cause more casualties when compared with open-air settings and cause fewer casualties when compared with closed-air settings. Leibovici and colleagues [13] compared four suicide bombings that occurred in Jerusalem from February 25, 1996 to March 4, 1996. Two were open-air explosions and two were bus explosions (closed settings). Of 204 casualties in open-air bombings, 15 died (7.8%), and of 93 patients injured in bus bombings, 46 died (49%), which demonstrates the severity of the bombings in closed settings. Almogy and colleagues [4] reported their experience with the Sbarro attack in August 2001 in Jerusalem, which happened in a crowed restaurant (semi-closed setting) and caused 146 casualties with 14 immediate deaths.

Injuries caused by bomb explosions are usually classified as primary, secondary, and tertiary blast injuries. The primary blast wounds are caused directly by the explosion after the sudden rise of pressure. Air-containing structures, such as lungs, middle ear, and gastrointestinal tract, are primarily injured. Although bowel perforation is rarely encountered (0–1.2%), Kluger [12] reported three cases in a suicide bombing in 2003.

Metal parts, bolts, and metal balls added by terrorists to the explosives cause secondary blast injuries. At the time of the explosions those metal parts are airborne and can cause superficial or deep tissue

wounds, depending on the proximity of the victims to the site of explosion. Tertiary blast injuries are caused when a victim is displaced by the blast and impacts against objects in proximity to the detonation, which results in multiple injuries and fractures of multiple bones. Fourth—or miscellaneous—blast injuries involve burns that result from burning clothes and close proximity to the enormously hot detonation site [11–13].

Maxillofacial injuries occur as result of second, third, and fourth blast-type injuries. Screws, metal bolts, and shrapnel that are attached to the explosives are displaced after the detonation and can injure the face, head, and neck [14]. Because these devices gain different types of energy after detonation, they also produce different types of injuries, some superficial and some deep. Life-threatening situations may occur after injury of major vessels in the neck by the metal parts. The intensity of the explosion causes other foreign bodies to be displaced. In one of the last suicide bombings, part of a watch was removed from a neck injury sustained by one of the victims. Soft tissue laceration also is present in the maxillofacial region after a blast. Some injuries are more severe than others, depending on the proximity of the injured person to the bomber at the time of explosion (Figs. 9, 10A–C). Hiss and colleagues [15] reported at least one case in which the cause of death was severe injury to the brain caused by shrapnel and screws, which discloses the lethal characteristics of these displaced metal devices. Zygomatic and mandibular bone fractures occur after the impact of displaced bolts and metal balls (secondary blast

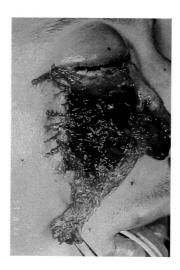

Fig. 9. Laceration of right portion of the face after an explosion. (Courtesy of C. Cohen, DMD, Caracas, Venezuela.)

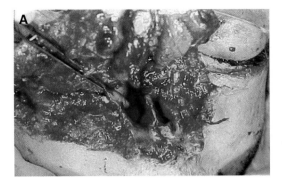
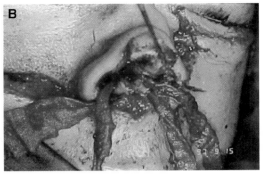
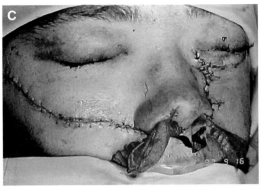

Fig. 10. (*A*) Severe soft tissue laceration after a suicide bombing. (*B*) Transoperative appearance. Note the insertion of iodoform gauze into the nasal area to sustained soft tissues. (*C*) Immediate postoperative appearance after suturing of wounds. (Courtesy of C. Cohen, DMD, Caracas, Venezuela.)

injury). Facial burns also occur as a result of the heat produced by the explosion.

## Summary

Oral and maxillofacial surgeons play an important role in the treatment of patients after terrorist attacks in Israel, because many wounded persons suffer from injuries to the facial area. Maxillofacial surgeons are part of the trauma team in most of the medical centers in the country and are called when a terrorist attack occurs. Because of the different types of weapons used by terrorists, different types of injuries are present, yet suicide bombers inflict the more vicious and unusual wounds.

## Acknowledgments

I would like to thank Prof. Dorrit W. Nitzan for her assistance in the surgical treatment of patients in Figs. 4A–D and 5. I also would like to thank Prof. Rephael Zeltser, Prof. Dorrit W. Nitzan, Prof. Joshua Lustmann, Prof. Arie Shteyer, Prof. Badri Azaz, and Dr. Shimon Shohat from the Department of Oral and Maxillofacial Surgery, Hadassah University Medical Center, Jerusalem, Israel, for their guidance and encouragement during my residency years at the department.

## References

[1] Adler J, Golan E, Golan J, et al. Terrorist bombing experience during 1975–79: casualties admitted to the Shaare Zedek Medical Center. Israel Journal of Medical Sciences 1983;19:189–93.
[2] Peleg K, Aharonson-Daniel L, Stein M, et al. Gunshot and explosion injuries: characteristics, outcomes and implications for care of terror-related injuries in Israel. Ann Surg 2004;239(3):311–8.
[3] Einav S, Feigenberg Z, Weisman C, et al. Evacuation priorities in mass casualty terror-related events: implications for contingency planning. Ann Surg 2004; 239(3):304–10.
[4] Almogy G, Belzberg H, Mintz Y, et al. Suicide

bombing attacks: update and modifications to the protocol. Ann Surg 2004;239(3):295–303.

[5] Heering SL, Shohat T, Lerman Y, et al. The epidemiology of injuries sustained by Israeli troops during the unrest in the territories administered by Israel, 1987–89. Israel Journal of Medical Sciences 1992;28:341–4.

[6] Nahlilei O, Baruchin AM, Neder A. Fractures of the mandible caused by stoning: return of an ancient entity. Trauma 1993;35(6):939–42.

[7] Hanoch J, Feigin E, Pikarsky A, et al. Stab wounds associated with terrorist activities in Israel. JAMA 1996;276(5):388–90.

[8] Robertson BC, Manson PN. High-energy ballistic and avulsive injuries: a management protocol for the next millennium. Surg Clin North Am 1999;79(6): 1489–502.

[9] Motamedi MHK. Primary management of maxillofacial hard and soft tissue gunshot and shrapnel injuries. J Oral Maxillofac Surg 2003;61(12):1390–8.

[10] Sadda RS. Maxillofacial war injuries during the Iraq-Iran war: an analysis of 300 cases. Int J Oral Maxillofac Surg 2003;32:209–14.

[11] Stein M, Hirshberg A. Medical consequences of terrorism: the conventional weapon threat. Surg Clin North Am 1999;79(6):1537–51.

[12] Kluger Y. Bomb explosions in acts of terrorism: detonation, wound ballistics, triage and medical concerns. Isr Med Assoc J 2003;5:235–40.

[13] Leibovici D, Gofrit ON, Stein M, et al. Blast injuries: bus versus open air bombings. A comparative study of injuries in survivors of open-air versus confined-space explosions. Trauma 1996;41(6):1030–5.

[14] Casapi N, Zeltser R, Regev A, et al. Maxillofacial gunshot injuries in hostility activities in 2000–2003. Refuat Hapeh Vehashinayim 2004;21(1):47–53.

[15] Hiss J, Freund M, Motro U, et al. The medico-legal investigation of the El Aqsah Intifada. Isr Med Assoc J 2002;4:549–53.

ELSEVIER
SAUNDERS

Oral Maxillofacial Surg Clin N Am 17 (2005) 281 – 287

**ORAL AND
MAXILLOFACIAL
SURGERY CLINICS**
of North America

# Improvised Explosive Devices and the Oral and Maxillofacial Surgeon

## Tamer Goksel, DDS, MD

*Oral and Maxillofacial Surgery Service, Brooke Army Medical Center, George C. Beach Avenue, San Antonio, TX 78234, USA*

Since 1983, Iraq has been involved in major conflicts, characterized by large-scale operations, against outside forces. Grenades, mortars, mines, and other explosive ordnance hazards can be found readily throughout this area of operation. Iraqi soldiers loyal to Saddam's Baath Party and members of the Sunni sect of Islam are modern insurgents and have the knowledge and experience in the use of these ordnance devices. It was during the Gulf War that the coalition forces first encountered improvised explosive devices (IEDs). Most such devices were set up in bunker complexes or were daisy chained with the attacks directed toward convoys (Fig. 1). Currently, IEDs pose the greatest threat to coalition convoys and are the major cause of US and coalition casualties.

During the current conflict and since the end of major operations, 40% to 60% of all attacks begin with an IED attack directed toward a convoy, a coalition checkpoint, or a high visibility civilian target [1]. After detonation of the IED, small arms fire directed toward vulnerable soft targets have become the normality. Most of these IEDs are remotely detonated using relatively low-technology devices, such as garage door openers, two-way radios, cellular phones, and pagers, to name a few [1]. As the name implies, an IED is an improvised device that is homemade and is designed to cause death or injury by using various explosive materials—commercial, military, or a combination of the two (Fig. 2). The

builder improvises not only with the materials at hand but also with the ever-changing fields of operation. Insurgents have managed to stay one step ahead of coalition efforts to neutralize their deadly efforts. IEDs are becoming more and more sophisticated and difficult to detect.

Three major types of IEDs are encountered in Iraq: package-type IEDs, vehicle-borne IEDs (VBIED), and suicide bomb IEDs [2]. They come in varying shapes and forms but have a few common components, including (1) a container, (2) an explosive fill, (3) a detonator, (4) a power supply to the detonator, and (5) a fuse [2].

The package-type IED consists mainly of mortar and artillery projectiles. Most of these military munitions are 60 mm or larger mortar and artillery rounds. They have been uncovered from roadway medians and manholes; they have been tossed from overpasses and hidden in underground maintenance passages. They have been found in soda cans and paper and plastic bags, and they have been contained in plaster objects made to look like concrete blocks, Meals Ready-To-Eat boxes, and dead animal carcasses found on roadsides.

VBIEDs use a vehicle as the container for the explosive device. The vehicles come in all shapes and sizes and have included donkey-drawn carts and ambulances. Depending on the size of the vehicle, the explosive charge has ranged from 100 to 1000 lb [3]. Mortar rounds, rocket warheads, C4 plastic explosives, and artillery rounds have been used in VBIEDs. Multiple vehicles commonly are used in a VBIED attack, in which a lead vehicle is used to breach a barrier or draw the attention of coalition forces. The explosive charged second vehicle is then detonated to inflict the greatest number of casualties.

The views and opinions expressed herein are those of the author and do not necessarily reflect those of the Department of Defense or the Department of the Army.

*E-mail address:* tamer.goksel@amedd.army.mil

1042-3699/05/$ – see front matter. Published by Elsevier Inc.
doi:10.1016/j.coms.2005.05.002

*oralmaxsurgery.theclinics.com*

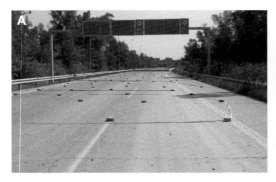 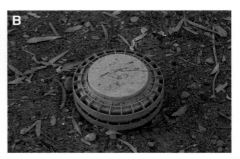

Fig. 1. (*A*) Daisy chained land mines on a major roadway. (*B*) A Singapore anti-tank land mine.

The suicide bomb IED is one of the most effective techniques in amassing mass casualties because the suicide bomber activates the detonation by hand. The explosives are hidden in vests, backpacks, and other clothing material. Vehicle-borne suicide bombers have greater accuracy and can inflict a high casualty ratio on their targets. Early detection of the threat and use of deadly force are the only options for neutralizing the bomber.

Coalition forces are constantly training and improvising their operational techniques to decrease the IED threat. Coalition convoy routes are easy to predict, and the surrounding urban terrain increases the vulnerability to enemy attacks. Coalition soldiers must keep a vigilant eye on subtle changes along the roadside. IED devices are usually placed during the hours of darkness and are detonated during high convoy traffic times, usually between 7:00 AM and 4:00 PM. Minor road obstacles, such as dirt, stone,

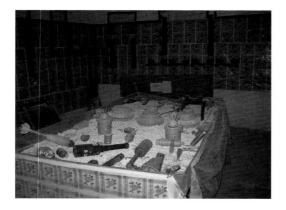

Fig. 2. Variety of uncovered and confiscated explosive devices.

and other debris, can be used to bottleneck vehicles to increase exposure time to the convoy. Patches of recently disturbed soil, vegetation piles of debris, or salvageable metal or wood left by the roadside should alert the convoy to a high level of threat. IEDs routinely are hidden in such objects. Some common convoy safety tips include varying vehicle speeds, vehicle distances, and vehicle numbers. Overwhelming firepower on several point and rear vehicles can be a significant deterrent. Once attacked, immediately engaging the enemy, refusing to stop in the kill zone, and minimizing the time spent in the ambush zone increase soldiers' survivability. Vehicle crews also should be vigilant when entering areas in which the locals are inexplicably absent and shops are closed for business during working hours.

IEDs have created a new class of casualties that presents a unique surgical challenge for oral and maxillofacial surgeons. The injury pattern and severity are much different from those seen in conventional trauma patients. Multiorgan systems are involved, which makes treatment-planning efforts difficult. Because of battlefield circumstances, patients are sometimes delayed significantly in their transport to a trauma center, and they frequently arrive at a trauma center with hypotension, hypothermia, and acidosis. Definitive care is delayed while the hemodynamic status and life-threatening injuries are stabilized. These patients need aggressive resuscitative efforts and require multiple surgical procedures. They have an increased mortality, which necessitates prolonged critical care services and an extended hospital stay and rehabilitative care. Because IEDs generally are detonated in areas to inflict high casualty ratios, mass casualty events at trauma centers are a common scenario. Hospital triage protocols must be well established in advance to prepare a timely response to the mass casualty event. Proper resource use is an ever-evolving challenge for hospital staff during these times.

Most (46%) casualties who presented to the combat support hospital in Baghdad, Iraq did were victims of IED and VBIED attacks. Other mechanisms of injury included non–battle-related injuries (18%), gunshot wounds (17%), mortar attacks (8%), motor vehicle crashes (8%), and rocket-propelled grenade attacks (8%). The statistics provided are the experiences of one Army oral and maxillofacial surgeon deployed to Operation Iraqi Freedom II from June 10, 2004 through December 15, 2004.

An IED induces four classes of injury. The primary blast injury is a result of the blast itself. The secondary blast injury is from the projectiles from the explosion. The tertiary blast injury results when the victim is thrust against stationary objects. The quaternary blast injury is from fire and heat generated by the explosion [4]. Penetrating, perforating, and avulsive fragmentation injuries are commonly seen in injuries that result from IEDs and VBIEDs.

The 31st Combat Support Hospital was located in the International Zone ("Green Zone") at the Ibn Sina Hospital in Baghdad, Iraq. This facility was the only head and neck trauma center for coalition forces in Iraq. The head and neck team at the facility consisted of two neurosurgeons, two oral and maxillofacial surgeons, and two ophthalmologists. Multiple teams were involved in the management of these complex surgical cases. A trauma surgeon was the lead surgical triage officer and was responsible for coordinating the surgical care of the patients. Advanced trauma life support protocols were used, and aggressive resuscitation and hemodynamic stability were the priority in the early management of these patients. An oral surgeon assisted in the early management of these patients by assessing the need for a surgical airway or assisting the anesthesiologist in securing a nonsurgical airway. Initial management of significant head and neck hemorrhage was controlled by local measures (eg, packing, direct pressure, suture ligation, clamping, electrocautery). Patients then were turned over to general or orthopedic surgery for stabilization of their urgent surgical needs. Surgical workload by service at the 31st Combat Support Hospital during this period was as follows: general surgery (40%), orthopedic surgery (36%), oral and maxillofacial surgery (8%), neurosurgery (6%), and other (10%). The "other" category consisted mainly of urologic and obstetric and gynecologic surgery.

Radiographic evaluation consisted of plain films in the trauma bay and CT evaluation as time and space allowed (Fig. 3). Not all maxillofacial injuries warranted CT imaging. All maxillofacial fragmenta-

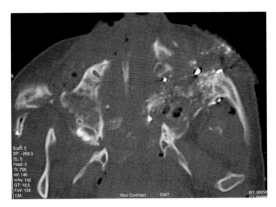

Fig. 3. Axial CT cut of fragmentation wound to midface.

tion wounds were imaged, however, to assess the location of fragments and evaluate the trajectory path in relation to vital structures. Some small entrance wounds resulted in devastating injuries caused by the velocity and trajectory of the projectile. Without the aid of radiographic imaging, ascertaining the location or the depth of injury caused by these fragments can be nearly impossible.

The need for a surgical airway was assessed early in the care of these patients. Injured patients frequently were transferred to a higher echelon of care for their definitive surgical needs. The higher echelon of care always was administered at distant sites, which necessitated air evacuation with several layovers before reaching a final destination. The transport time interval between leaving the combat support hospital and arriving at the final destination could last 10 to 15 days. Any patient with an airway concern, including orally and nasally intubated patients with the probability of endotracheal tube displacement, were provided with a surgical airway (tracheostomy). Patients with panfacial trauma, severe midfacial fractures, prolonged intubation, and multisystemic trauma that necessitated return trips to the operating room were provided with a tracheostomy before mobilization to the next echelon of care. All cricothyrotomies were converted to tracheostomy before transport.

All fragmentation injuries were considered contaminated (Fig. 4). Commonly, large surface areas of skin were peppered with dirt, gravel, grass, wood, plastic, car seat foam, and other organic materials. Prophylactic antibiotics and tetanus prophylaxis was administered to patients on admission. In the operating room setting, a pulsed lavage system with a high volume of sterile saline was used. This process was followed by meticulous débridement and gauze sponge wound cleansing using a dilute povidone-

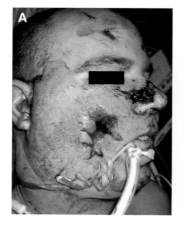
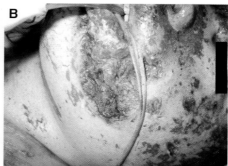

Fig. 4. (*A*) Fragmentation wounds to face after VBIED attack. (*B*) Fragmentation wound to face after detonation of roadside IED.

iodine solution. Superficial wounds were débrided thoroughly and closed primarily. Wounds that were too deep to débride effectively were packed with iodoform or regular gauze, however. All wounds were handled gently, and soft tissue débridement and sacrifice were kept to a minimum. Dead spaces were eliminated with deep resorbable sutures, and the dermis was everted with subcuticular sutures for a tension-free closure. Prolene sutures were used to re-approximate skin edges.

When IEDs and VBIEDs are involved, patients should be assessed for burn-related injuries (Fig. 5). One should look for soot in the nares and oral cavity, perform a direct laryngoscopy to inspect for upper airway edema, and maintain a low threshold for endotracheal intubation. When in doubt, intubate. In short order, the rapidly ensuing oropharyngeal edema makes securing the airway a much greater challenge.

The endotracheal tube can be secured to the upper dentition with 24-gauge circumdental wiring. This method is much gentler on the burn-affected soft tissues. Once the airway is secured, one should evaluate the orbits for compartment syndrome secondary to the periorbital edema. Have a low threshold to perform a lateral canthotomy and cantholysis to relieve orbital pressure. With a secure airway and protected globes, attention can be directed to wound débridement. Gentle wound débridement with sterile saline and gauze is effective. After thorough débridement, apply bacitracin to the head and neck region and ophthalmic bacitracin to the periorbita. Because of its caustic effects on the eyes, silvadene and other commonly used burn ointments should not be used on the face.

Maxillofacial fractures are not life-threatening injuries, and definitive care can be delayed until a

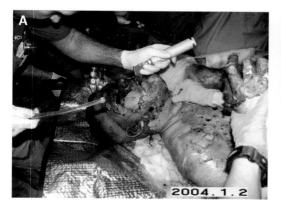
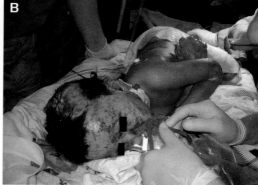

Fig. 5. (*A*) Airway evaluation in burn patients. (*B*) Facial burns caused by explosions.

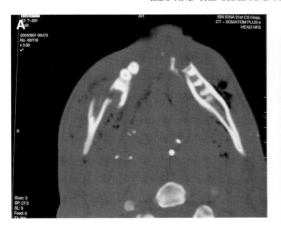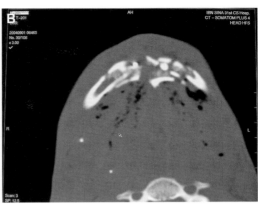

Fig. 6. (*A*) Flail mandibular segment. (*B*) A lower axial CT of the same patient.

patient is hemodynamically stable and the more urgent issues are addressed. The exception to this rule is a flail mandibular segment that compromises the airway (Fig. 6). For flail segments, the treatment involves establishing a surgical airway or stabilizing the segments by an external fixation device or an open reduction internal fixation technique. During the early healing phase, time allows the injured soft and hard tissues to declare their vitality. Conservative débridement of the soft and hard tissues at the combat support hospital level allows an adequate time to elapse for the tissues to declare themselves. Treatment options for mandibular fractures at the combat support hospital include (1) skeletal fixation using surgical wires, (2) maxillomandibular fixation using arch bars and circumdental wires, and (3) external fixation using the Joe-Hall Morris appliance or the Hoffman II orthopedic wrist appliance (Figs. 7 and 8). Primary reconstruction with bone plates and screws in the austere combat environment yield poor results fraught with infections and plate exposures. Re-evaluation and treatment planning

of complex facial fractures with the aid of three-dimensional CT reconstruction (Fig. 9) and stereolithography can enhance surgical outcomes greatly.

In severe midface fractures, as with mandibular fractures, the primary concern is the patency of the airway. Because of transportation issues addressed earlier, a low threshold is kept in obtaining a surgical airway. A tracheostomy alleviates the need to manipulate the injured oral and nasal cavities and provides a better opportunity to maintain pulmonary toiletry. All facial fractures that involve the orbits require an ophthalmologic consultation. A surgeon always should evaluate the orbits for a compartment syndrome as a result of bony impingement or a retrobulbar hematoma. One should maintain a low tolerance in performing lateral canthotomy and cantholysis if the need should arise. Midface fractures caused by IEDs or VBIEDs result in wounds

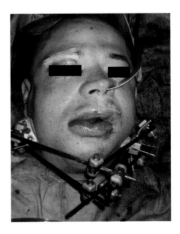

Fig. 8. External fixation using the Hoffman II wrist appliance.

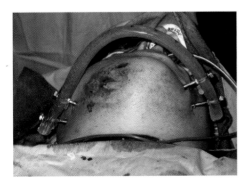

Fig. 7. External fixation using the Joe-Hall Morris appliance.

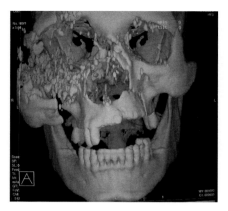

Fig. 9. Three-dimensional CT reconstruction of gunshot wound to face.

that are grossly contaminated with metallic fragments, rocks, dirt, and other organic materials. The paranasal sinuses are obliterated with contaminants, secretions, and blood. Thorough and meticulous irrigation and débridement must be accomplished. Because of the nature of the injuries, patients usually undergo operations on numerous occasions by various specialists. Coordinating efforts with the other surgical specialties provides oral and maxillofacial surgeons many opportunities to evaluate and redébride wounds. Initial management of maxillary fractures at the combat support hospital level included skeletal fixation using surgical wires and external fixation using the Hoffman II wrist appliance in severely comminuted midface fractures (Fig. 10). Conservative tissue management, serial irrigations and débridement, and fracture stabilization with external fixation or skeletal fixation techniques yielded the most favorable results.

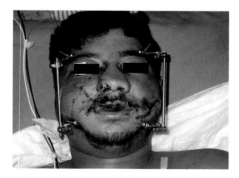

Fig. 10. Skeletal fixation of midface fractures using the Hoffman II appliance.

**Box 1. Lessons learned**

Maxillofacial fragmentation injuries of any size should undergo CT scanning

Patients who have panfacial trauma, severe midface fractures, prolonged intubation, and multisystemic trauma that requires numerous trips to the operating room should undergo a tracheostomy during initial surgery

Deep, penetrating wounds that are difficult to débride adequately should be packed

Superficial wounds and wounds that are débrided effectively should be closed primarily when possible

Victims of IED or VBIED should be evaluated for airway burns and intubated before ensuing upper airway edema

Patients who have facial burn should be evaluated for orbital compartment syndrome, and canthotomy and cantholysis should be performed before ensuing periorbital edema

Patients who have head and neck burns should have an endotracheal tube secured to the dentition with circumdental wires

Hard and soft tissue débridement and periosteal stripping should be kept to a minimum until a wound declares itself

The surgeon should stabilize flail mandibular segments by fixation techniques or secure the airway by tracheostomy or endotracheal intubation

The surgeon should obtain an ophthalmologic consultation when facial fractures involve the orbits, evaluate the globes for compartment syndrome, and perform canthotomy/cantholysis as necessary

One should evaluate midface injuries for septal hematomas and drain and support them as indicated

Craniofacial plating should not be used in contaminated wounds or wounds with large soft tissue defects

Box 1 contains a summary of lessons learned from experience at combat support hospitals.

## References

[1] Pike J. Improvised explosive devices (IEDs): Iraq. Available at: www.globalsecurity.org. Accessed February 15, 2005.

[2] Pike J. Improvised explosive devices (IEDs): booby traps. Available at: www.globalsecurity.org. Accessed February 15, 2005.

[3] Pike J. Vehicle borne IEDs (VBIEDs). Available at: www.globalsecurity.org. Accessed February 15, 2005.

[4] Kluger Y, Peleg K, Daniel-Aharonson L, et al. The special injury pattern in terrorist bombings. J Am Coll Surg 2004;199:875–9.

ELSEVIER
SAUNDERS

Oral Maxillofacial Surg Clin N Am 17 (2005) 289–298

ORAL AND
MAXILLOFACIAL
SURGERY CLINICS
of North America

# Radiation Injuries, Triage, and Treatment after a Nuclear Terrorist Attack

Robert K. McGhee, DDS*, Daron C. Praetzel, DMD,
Christopher C. Medley, DDS, MD

*Department of Oral and Maxillofacial Surgery, Wilford Hall Medical Center, 2200 Bergquist Drive, Suite 1,
Lackland Air Force Base, TX 78236-9908, USA*

Oral and maxillofacial surgeons are comfortable treating patients in a trauma setting, whether in a small local hospital or in a major metropolitan level 1 trauma center. Maxillofacial trauma care remains a core component of our specialty. How does our role change in a mass disaster scenario that involves radiologic weaponry? How do we fit into the disaster response team to provide much needed maxillofacial trauma care and what are the risks to us, as providers, when treating these patients? Oral and maxillofacial surgeons must be knowledgeable of the effects of radiation exposure and protective measures to limit that exposure for patients and health care personnel. We must be able to prioritize care through triage and alter our treatment modalities when dealing with this unique type of injury. The ability to manage radiologic injuries has become an essential component to add to our core competencies.

## Sources of radiation attack

Radiologic contamination from a terrorist attack may come from several different routes, three of which are discussed most often. The first is a nuclear attack from outside our borders. Weapons of this type carry a large destructive capacity but require significant resources and technical support to make such a device viable. The capability of such a strike is only possible by technologically advanced nations, and the probability of an intercontinental strike currently is low.

The second terrorist route involves an attack on a source of radiation already present within our borders. Nuclear power plants within the United States provide a ready-made target. With continued planning by terrorist networks to breach security efforts at these facilities, this type of attack is considered much more probable than a conventional missile attack. An attack on a power plant could be performed by smaller numbers of individuals and with less financial backing than a missile attack.

The third possible option for terrorists is the radiologic dispersal device, which is frequently referred to as a "dirty bomb." Such a weapon involves a small amount of explosives packaged with radioactive material. This radioactive material can be found in hospitals, research laboratories, and construction sites [1]. The radiologic dispersal device is designed to instill panic among the public with the fear of radioactive contamination. It is probable that the level of radiation used would be minimal, based on the logistics of creating such a bomb [1]. The risk of cancer or lasting injury to the public or treatment team likely would be small in an event that involved a radiologic dispersal device [2]. These dirty bombs, sometimes referred to as "suitcase bombs," should be considered and managed more like traditional explo-

The opinions expressed in this article are those of the authors and do not reflect the views of the United States Air Force.

* Corresponding author.
*E-mail address:* robert.mcghee@lackland.af.mil (R.K. McGhee).

sive devices. Blast injuries are the most commonly treated injury, but psychological effects may be far reaching [1].

## Radiation facts

Radiation exposure is expressed in Gray (Gy) or Sieverts (Sv). The older units for these are rad and rem. 1 Gray equals 100 rad, and 1 Sievert equals 100 rem. Relative hazard approximations are presented in Table 1 [3]. The amount of radioactive contamination is measured in units of Bequerels (Bq) (1 disintegration/sec). Total exposure is based on the principles of time, distance, and shielding. Radiation dose is decreased by reducing the time spent in the radiation area (moderately effective), increasing the distance from a radiation source (very effective), or using metal or concrete shielding (less practical). Radiation is colorless, odorless, tasteless, and invisible. The only way to determine whether radioactive material is present is to perform radiologic surveys with specialized equipment [4]. Dosing to personnel who respond first to a scene after a radiologic event can be much higher than for later arrivals. Appropriate dose-rate meters must be available to determine the exposure accurately.

## Risk to health care providers

There have been no reports of health care providers ever suffering radiation injury while perform-

Table 1
Approximation of the relative hazard

| Dose | Relative hazard |
| --- | --- |
| Approximately 10 mGy or 10 mSv (1 Gy or rem) or less | No acute effects and only a small chance of subsequent cancer |
| Approximately 0.1 Gy or 0.1 Sv | No acute effects; subsequent additional risk of cancer approximately 0.5% |
| Approximately 1 Gy or 1 Sv | Nausea, vomiting possible, mild bone marrow depression, subsequent risk of cancer 5% |
| >2 Gy or Sv | Definite nausea, vomiting, medical evaluation, and treatment required |

*Data from* Department of Homeland Security Working Group on Radiological Dispersal Device Preparedness. Medical guidelines for ionizing radiation and terrorist incidents: important points for the patient and you. Washington, DC: Department of Homeland Security; 2003.

ing basic life support on an exposed or contaminated patient. Protection for providers is best accomplished by observing standard precautions, including wearing a mask, gloves, and protective clothing. Care of life-threatening injuries should not be delayed because of possible radiation exposure. The primary concern for providers as they approach the site of a radiologic event should be the degree and type of injuries among the patients. Life-threatening injuries should be treated immediately. More time and caution may be taken with victims whose injuries are less severe, which is explained in more detail in the triage section of this article.

Nuclear detonation, or explosion at a nuclear reactor, is likely to spread over a large area. The precautions for providers are essentially the same, however. There are three points of concern for providers as they reach a potentially contaminated disaster site: (1) immediate care of victims with life-threatening injuries, (2) respiratory protection for health care providers, and (3) skin protection for health care providers.

Contaminated personnel, equipment, and vehicles can be cleaned later, after the acute traumatic injuries have been addressed. Three levels of protective masks are available for personal protection equipment. Radiologic events require "Level C" protection, which is the lowest protection level available. Numerous types of masks are available, ranging from masks that are fit-tested, cartridge-filtered respirators to masks that are high-efficiency particulate air filter masks to ordinary surgical masks. These masks provide good protection against particulate inhalation. Sites suspected of contamination with radiologic material also may be suspected of chemical or biologic contamination. Masks equipped to protect against these agents likewise protect against radiologic contamination. Protection of the skin of health care providers is easily accomplished by wearing simple protective items readily available to all oral and maxillofacial surgeons. Normal barrier clothing and gloves found in an office setting, emergency department, or operating room provide excellent protection. Other hazards may drive the choice of protective wear. Protective clothing designed for fire, heat, or chemicals more than adequately protect health care providers against radioactive contamination.

## Decontamination of patients

An initial fear of patient contamination may affect decisions of the attending treatment team. Studies show that the "levels of intrinsic radiation within the patient" are not of a significant amount to be a threat to the medical staff [5]. The medical staff should concern themselves first with life-saving therapies, because decontamination may be performed after stabilization of a patient [6]. Surgical attire such as gown, mask, gloves, caps, eye protection, and shoe covers helps minimize exposure [1]. A dosimeter also should be given to each member of the team to monitor exposure levels.

The priority in decontamination should be caring for open wounds. It is important to mention that immediate care should focus primarily on preventing internal contamination. Skin or wound contamination is almost never immediately life threatening; the priority is placed on treating conventional trauma injuries. After patient stabilization, steps should be taken to determine if internal contamination has occurred. Nasal swabs of both nares should be obtained as soon as possible, as should urine and feces specimens, which aid in determining whether internal contamination has occurred [3]. The characteristics of a wound affect the absorption and decontamination process. Abrasions disrupt the skin barrier and increase the absorption potential. Contaminants are usually easily accessible in abrasion injuries and are easy to decontaminate. The areas should be irrigated copiously with saline for several minutes [5]. Lacerations are more difficult than surface abrasions to decontaminate. These injuries require decontamination through surgical excision. Puncture wounds are the most difficult to decontaminate because of the difficulty in determining the depth and degree of the contamination and poor accessibility. Water picks and pulsating water irrigation systems have been used successfully in the past [3].

Removal of a patient's clothing can reduce contamination by 70% to 90% [6]. Patients should be washed with soap and water after clothing removal, with special attention paid to the exposed skin areas. Soap is 95% effective because soap emulsifies and dissolves contamination. One should use commercial shampoo for hair decontamination. Hair conditioner or shampoo that contains conditioners should not be used because of its ability to bind to the hair proteins. This binding makes it more difficult to remove the contaminants. Hair may need to be cut to remove the contaminants fully [3]. Recommended cleaning solutions for skin and wounds are soap and water, normal saline, povidone-iodine and water, and hexachlorophene 3% detergent cleanser and water. Ideally, decontamination takes place on the way to the hospital or outside the hospital in a decontamination area [1,5].

A radiation dosimeter is a portable device used to measure the amount of radiation contamination present in a given source. Radiation meters should be used when available to guide the decontamination process. It may be difficult to remove all of the contamination; decontaminating to a level that is two times the background radiation level should be adequate. Decontamination efforts should be stopped if the goal is not reached after the third attempt or when further decontamination attempts are seen to reduce the contamination by less than 10%. It is critical to be consistent with the device-to-skin distance to decrease survey error. It is important not to cause unnecessary damage to the skin while removing skin contamination. The stratum corneum of the epithelium is replaced every 12 to 15 days. Consequently, contaminants that are not removed and not absorbed by the body are sloughed off within 2 weeks of exposure.

## Triage of patients

Military physicians—and many other physicians—long have emphasized triage as a way to organize the chaos of a mass casualty. Triage for radiation injury patients is different from triage for conventionally injured patients. The radiation injury may not be manifested until days to weeks after exposure. Radiation injury triage is primarily based on a patient's conventional injuries and then is modified by radiation injury level. One triage system that may be used divides patients into four categories (Box 1) [7]. The delayed patient requires treatment but the injuries are not immediately life threatening. The immediate patient requires swift intervention to prevent loss of life. The minimal patient has minor injuries that often can be managed by ancillary personnel or self-care. The expectant patient is not likely to survive regardless of medical intervention. A preliminary assessment of the level of radiation injury is made for patients with exposure symptoms, such as nausea, vomiting, diarrhea, fever, ataxia, seizures, prostration, and hypotension [7].

The triage usually takes place in a holding area near the hospital. The evaluation is quick, with checks of respiration, cardiovascular function, mental status, and extent of injury. The quick check allows one provider—the triage officer—to move among patients and make decisions as to which patients will benefit most from treatment. It is necessary to assess traumatic injury and medical conditions before consideration of radiation exposure. Time to vomiting is an important assessment that must be made.

---

**Box 1. Radiation triage classification**

**Delayed:** Casualty with only radiation injury, without gross neurological symptoms (ataxia, seizures, impaired cognition). For trauma combined with radiation injury, all surgical procedures must be completed within 36–48 hours of radiation exposure, or delayed until at least 2 months after the injury.

**Immediate:** Those requiring immediate lifesaving intervention. Pure radiation injury is not acutely life-threatening unless the irradiation is massive. If a massive dose has been received, the patient is classified as Expectant.

**Minimal:** Buddy care is particularly useful here. Casualties with radiological injury should have all wounds and lacerations meticulously cleaned and then closed.

**Expectant:** Receive appropriate supportive treatment compatible with resources large doses of analgesics as needed.

*Data from* Radiological injuries. In: Szul A, editor. Emergency war surgery. Chapter 30. Washington (DC): Library of Congress Cataloging-in-Publication Data, Borden Institute; 2004. p. 30.1–30.7.

---

When the time to vomiting is less than 4 hours, a patient should be referred for immediate evaluation. When the time to vomiting is more than 4 hours, a patient can be referred for delayed evaluation (24–72 hours), assuming that there are no concurrent injuries. Patients who experience radiation-induced emesis within 1 hour after a radiation exposure require extensive and prolonged medical intervention. These patients typically do not survive the radiation injury [3]. Cardiopulmonary resuscitation is not initiated during the triage phase.

Thermal burns are encountered during this tasking. Patients with burns that involve less than 20% of the total body surface area should be treated as outpatients in a mass casualty. Hospitalization should be reserved for patients with burns over 20% to 50% of the body. Persons with burns over more than 50% of the body should be treated only when health care personnel ascertain that resources are available. Patients in this category have a particularly bad prognosis, especially in a mass casualty scenario. Burns to sensitive areas such as the head and neck,

the hands or feet will require hospitalization even if they involve less than 20% of the body area. [1,5]

**Nuclear weapon injuries**

Review of the injuries from nuclear or radiological weapons reveals four main types of injury. They can be called the "Damaging Factors of Nuclear Explosion." [4] and include: Light Radiation, Shock Wave, Penetrating Radiation, and Radioactive Contamination.

*Light radiation injuries (Thermal Burns)*

A fireball is formed upon initial detonation of a nuclear weapon resulting in superheating of anything nearby. This rapid increase of temperature results in the production of intense light and thermal radiation, which may produce burns of severe intensity, even at great distances. Many burn casualties should be expected from a nuclear detonation and may overwhelm treatment facilities Rapidly [5,8].

The severity of a burn depends on the strength of the source of light radiation, the proximity to that source, and the protective properties of the clothing worn by the burn victim [4]. Exposed areas of the head and neck may be particularly vulnerable in the general public during an attack. Although burn injuries are discussed elsewhere in this issue, immediate care to burn patients in this scenario follows a step-by-step process:

1. Stop the burning
2. Ensure airway patency and control hemorrhage
3. Remove all constricting articles (eg, rings, boots, watches, belts)
4. Cover a patient to preserve body temperature and prevent gross contamination
5. Establish intravenous access and begin resuscitation with lactated Ringer's solution

The light radiation may have a burning or blinding effect on the eyes, which may be especially problematic if the attack occurs during a time when the eyes are accustomed to low light levels (ie, at night or during twilight). Burns may occur to the eyelids, the cornea, or the retina [4]. Burns associated with radiation exposure have a much higher mortality rate than normal thermal burns. Researchers have proposed that radiation-induced bone marrow suppression and infections are responsible for the increased mortality [7].

*Shock wave (blast injury)*

The blast from a detonation may result in severe injuries that are more familiar to trauma surgeons or maxillofacial surgeons. Shock wave injuries can be subdivided into four categories: primary, secondary, tertiary, and miscellaneous.

Primary injuries are often called "direct injuries" and result from the overpressure released at detonation. The air-filled cavities, such as lungs, ears, and gastrointestinal tract, are at particular risk. Oral and maxillofacial surgeons may be the first to make this diagnosis. During a head and neck examination for facial trauma, examination of the ear includes visualization of the tympanic membrane. Rupture of the tympanic membrane may be the first sign of an overpressure injury. Many patients who are close enough to a nuclear blast to receive this type of injury do not survive the thermal burn because of proximity to the source [1,5].

Secondary injuries are "indirect injuries" and result from flying debris. The shock wave production is associated with formation of an overpressure wave with high winds. These winds initially move outward from the source and then reverse direction briefly. The resulting winds can turn ordinary ground debris and glass into missile-like projectiles and may cause various types of blunt or penetrating injuries. These winds may be strong enough to move automobiles or even larger objects [7]. Injuries from flying debris may occur more frequently in the head and neck region, because these areas are often unprotected [1,5,8]. Isolated facial fractures, lacerations, and avulsions of soft tissue can be seen with smaller flying debris from low-energy events. Crush injuries and panfacial fractures are more likely in larger, high-energy explosions.

Tertiary injuries are seen when people are actually picked up and thrown by the winds or explosion. The resulting injuries are those typically experienced in a trauma bay from motor vehicle accidents or falls [1]. Fractures of the facial skeleton may be seen with injuries of either the secondary or tertiary type. Miscellaneous injuries represent any other injuries associated with the blast that are not otherwise categorized. One example involves injuries to people that result from the collapse of a building [1].

*Penetrating radiation*

The third damaging factor of a nuclear explosion is penetrating radiation. Two important types of radiation released are electromagnetic (gamma) radiation and particulate (alpha, beta, and neutron) radiation. Regular clothing acts as a shield and prevents alpha particles from damaging the victim. Protection from beta particles requires more significant shielding, such as a solid wall. Gamma and neutron radiation are the most active biologically and are the most significant components of penetrating radiation. Lead shielding is required to protect against gamma and neutron radiation. Whole-body radiation results in

Table 2
Acute radiation syndrome (whole body or extensive partial body)

| Dose | Clinical status | Description |
|------|-----------------|-------------|
| 0–1 Gy | Generally Asymptomatic | White blood count normal or minimally depressed below baseline levels at 3–5 weeks after the accident |
| 1–8 Gy | Hematopoetic syndrome | Main prodromal signs and symptoms include anorexia, nausea, vomiting, and (occasionally) skin erythema, fever, mucositis, and diarrhea; laboratory analysis in cases with whole-body exposure >2 Gy can show an initial granulocytosis, with pancytopenia evident 20–30 days after the accident; subsequent systemic effects of the hematologic phase of acute radiation syndrome include immunodysfunction, increased infectious complications, possible hemorrhage, sepsis, anemia, and impaired wound healing |
| 8–30 Gy | Gastrointestinal syndrome | Symptoms may include early, severe nausea, vomiting, and watery diarrhea, often within hours after the accident; in severe cases, the patient may present with shock and possibly renal failure and cardiovascular collapse; death from gastrointestinal syndrome usually occurs 8–14 days after the accident; hematopoietic syndrome occurs concomitantly |
| >20 Gy | Cardiovascular/ central nervous syndrome | Patients may experience a burning sensation within the first hour after accident, prostration, and neurologic signs of ataxia and confusion; death is inevitable and usually occurs within 24–48 hours |

*Data from* Department of Homeland Security Working Group on Radiological Dispersal Device Preparedness. Medical guidelines for ionizing radiation and terrorist incidents: important points for the patient and you. Washington, DC: Department of Homeland Security; 2003.

radiation sickness and can be lethal in a matter of days if left untreated [5]. Multiple manifestations of radiation sickness are seen in proportion to the dosage of radiation received and are summarized in Table 2 [5].

Neurovascular syndrome is the most severe manifestation of radiation sickness and results from the highest dose of radiation exposure (>3000 cGy). To receive this much radiation, a patient would have to be close to the detonation site. Few patients who present to emergency rooms after nuclear attack present with this syndrome, because few would survive the initial detonation. These patients may become ataxic or convulsive. This level of radiation exposure progresses quickly to respiratory depression, coma, and, ultimately, death [5].

Gastrointestinal syndrome is seen in relatively small numbers after a nuclear attack because patients typically do not survive their other, more severe, concomitant injuries. They must have received more than 1000 cGy of radiation and generally develop bloody diarrhea 4 to 5 days after exposure. They have a decrease in lymphocytes and platelets and are subsequently at increased risk for infections and hemorrhage, which may prove fatal [5].

Patients who have hematopoietic syndrome have received a range of radiation exposure (generally <1000 cGy), and the degree of bone marrow suppression depends on the total dose. Generally, the syndrome begins 2 to 3 weeks after exposure. Patients begin to develop increased bleeding tendencies with potential for uncontrolled hemorrhage. As bleeding continues, decreased resistance to infection occurs.

All of the radiation sickness syndromes show an initial nonspecific response with a latent phase that follows. The initial nonspecific symptoms include malaise, weakness, anorexia, vomiting, and diarrhea. The latent period varies based on the severity of the exposure. The neurovascular syndrome may have an extremely fast latent phase. The latent period is a relative "feel good" period [5]. Signs and symptoms of radiation sickness are outlined in Table 3.

*Radioactive contamination (fall out)*

The residual radiation that exists after the first minute of a nuclear detonation is considered fall out. The amount of this radiation varies and immediately begins to decay. The farther the distance from the detonation site and the longer the time since detonation, the smaller the radiation fall out is in a specific area. Radiation fall out contributes to the total body radiation exposure and the resulting radiation sickness as described previously [5].

**Treatment considerations**

The nuclear battlefield is a unique scenario that has many complicating factors. Any of the previously described injuries alone can be devastating. In combination, however, they act synergistically to increase the overall morbidity and mortality of victims [5,6]. After the detonation of a nuclear device, most of casualties demonstrate injuries that consist of a combination of radiologic injury, thermal injury, and blast injury. The treatment of these combined injuries requires a modification from the normal treatment of any single type of injury. Many injuries that otherwise would be easily survivable become potentially life threatening.

Estimated reported combined injuries from Hiroshima and Nagasaki were as follows [6]: burn and wound and radiation, 20%; burn and radiation, 40%; mechanical and radiation, 5%; other, 35%. The victims of the atomic blasts in Japan developed significant complications 2 to 3 weeks after exposure to hematopoietic depressive levels of radiation. The

Table 3
Medical aspects of radiation injuries

| Probability/degree of exposure | Signs and symptoms | | | | | | |
|---|---|---|---|---|---|---|---|
| | Nausea | Vomiting | Diarrhea | Hyperthermia | Erythema | Hypotension | CNS dysfunction |
| Unlikely | − | − | − | − | − | − | − |
| Probable | ++ | + | +/− | +/− | − | − | − |
| Severe | +++ | +++ | +/+++ | +/+++ | −/++ | +/++ | −/++ |

*Abbreviation:* CNS, central nervous system.
*Data from* Borden Institute. Radiologic injuries: emergency war surgery. Washington, DC: Walter Reed Army Medical Center; 2004.

treating physicians witnessed a slowdown, or cessation, of wound healing. They saw an increased incidence in hemorrhage and infection [6]. Multiple studies quoted by Conklin and colleagues [6] cited the animal research that shows that the mortality of a wound increases when inflicted after a dose of radiation. This decrease in healing also applies to hard tissues, which has been shown in rabbit studies, in which double the healing time was seen for fractured bones after radiation exposure. Studies have indicated that a latent phase, immediately after radiation exposure, exists when wound healing may be unhindered [6].

Whenever possible, surgical therapy should be performed within 36 hours after radiation exposure. This approach takes advantage of the latent phase. Otherwise, surgery should be delayed 6 to 8 weeks after exposure to allow the body's healing capacity to regenerate to whatever degree it can [5]. This approach has direct implications for oral and maxillofacial surgeons. Quick stabilization or reduction of fractures is critical for providing the best opportunity for healing. Delayed reduction of fractures may result in non-union or infection. If early stabilization is performed, further reconstruction or repair may be performed in a more controlled setting 6 to 8 weeks later.

Another modification is recommended after review of traditional battlefield therapies. Historically, a wound suffered in combat was stabilized and left open. Injuries exposed to radiation pose more risk of infection if left open to heal by secondary intention, however. A wound exposed to radiation should be closed rather than left open, and it should be accomplished within 36 to 48 hours [7]. Combined injuries are further manifested by the radiation effects on the gastrointestinal tract. The alteration to the mucosal lining affects the absorption of medications. This action alters drug metabolism, which could lead to toxic dosages being inadvertently administered.

Medical countermeasures have been developed over several years to help prevent or limit some of the sequelae associated with radiation exposure. Use of specific agents or drugs requires knowledge of the type of radiation exposure. All treatments do not fit all situations, and some have significant side effect profiles. The following countermeasures should be considered after a radiologic event.

*Amifostine*

Amifostine is a phosphorylated aminothiol use as a protective agent for radiation exposure. When taken 15 to 30 minutes before radiation exposure, amifostine acts as a free radical scavenger that protects cell membranes and DNA against radiation-induced free radicals. It has been shown to decrease radiation toxicity in patients who are receiving radiotherapy. Its intravenous use has been limited by its severe side effects, however. Subcutaneous administration is being investigated and may limit side effects. The idea of giving amifostine to first responders who must go to a radiation site is currently being investigated [3].

*Bicarbonate (NAHCO$_3$)*

The treatment of choice for a radiologic event that involves uranium is bicarbonate. Bicarbonate is readily available and is well known to most providers who respond to radiologic incidents. One of the main risks of uranium exposure is acute tubular necrosis, which may be prevented by urine alkalinization. Bicarbonate should be administered either through the oral or intravenous route, and urine pH should be followed frequently to ensure alkalinity. Alkaline urine forms a nontoxic uranium carbonate complex that is promptly excreted by the kidney [3].

*Colony-stimulating factors (cytokines)*

Cytokines are naturally occurring glycoproteins that induce bone marrow stem cells to proliferate and differentiate into a wide variety of mature cell types. Colony-stimulating factors act on hematopoietic cells by binding to cell surface receptors, which stimulate proliferation, differentiation, commitment, and end-cell functional activation [3]. This class of medications is currently used for decreasing the infection rate and increasing neutrophil recovery in patients who have neutropenia. Currently, the use of these medications in a patient population exposed to radiation is not approved by the US Food and Drug Administration, but off-label use may be considered by providers on a case-by-case basis [3].

*Diethylenetriaminepenta-acetate*

Diethylenetriaminepenta-acetate is one of the chelating agents. The mechanism of action involves exchanging calcium for another metal, such as plutonium or americium. Once these metals are chelated, they are excreted much more easily. This therapy has been in use for 40 years with good success rates and few adverse reactions. In an emergency exposure setting, administration should begin within 6 hours of exposure. Development of an oral form of this medication would make access easier in a mass casualty event [3].

Table 4
Threshold thyroid radioactive exposures and recommended doses of potassium iodide for different risk groups

| Age groups | Predicted thyroid exposures (cGy) | Potassium iodide dose (mg) | Number of 130-mg tablets | Number of 65-mg tablets |
|---|---|---|---|---|
| Adults over 40 years | ≥500 | | | |
| Adults 18–40 years | ≥10 | | | |
| Pregnant or lactating women | | 130 | 1 | 2 |
| Adolescents 12–18 years[a] | ≥5 | 65 | 1/2 | 1 |
| Children 3–12 years | | | | |
| >1 month through 3 years | | 32 | 1/4 | 1/2 |
| Birth through 1 month | | 16 | 1/8 | 1/4 |

[a] Adolescents approaching adult size (>70 kg) should receive the full adult dose (130 mg).
*Data from* Department of Homeland Security Working Group on Radiological Dispersal Device Preparedness. Medical guidelines for ionizing radiation and terrorist incidents: important points for the patient and you. Washington, DC: Department of Homeland Security; 2003.

*Potassium iodide*

Potassium iodide is the treatment of choice for prevention of uptake of radiologic material by the thyroid gland (Table 4). Potassium iodide is useful only for protecting the thyroid; it is not a generic anti-radiation medicine, as is often popularized by the media [3]. It must be taken before exposure or within a few hours after exposure. Twenty-four hours after exposure, potassium iodide is only 7% effective. Questions exist about the usefulness of potassium iodide in patients older than age 40 [3]. Recommended dosing for potassium iodide is seen in Table 4.

*Prussian blue*

Prussian blue has been used in prior radiologic events. It is effective in helping the body to excrete isotopes of cesium and thallium. Prussian blue has a high affinity for cesium and thallium and, when taken orally, it sequesters these isotopes in the gut. This action increases the fecal excretion of the isotopes. The biologic half-life of thallium and cesium is significantly reduced after Prussian blue administration. It was used in Goiania, Brazil in 1987 in 46 patients and was successful in reducing the half-life of isotopes on average from 39 days to 16 days. There is currently a limited supply of Prussian blue in the United States, and the only supplier is in Germany. This factor could delay delivery times of large quantities to 12 to 18 months in the event of a mass casualty or multiple simultaneous events [3].

*Stem cell transplantation*

Stem cell transplantation is a controversial therapy for persons exposed to large doses of radiation. As the level of radiation exposure increases, the number of hematopoietic cells in the marrow decreases. The radiation level that causes irreversible failure of the hematopoietic system varies. When serious damage occurs to the hematopoietic system, any surviving stem cells can migrate to the damaged areas and repopulate the entire system. This is the basis of the transplant. When a marrow or stem cell transplant is performed between monozygotic twins, hematopoiesis is safely restored. Not everyone has an identical twin, however, and significant immunosuppression may be required to prevent graft-versus-host disease when a nonidentical host is used. To this point, few transplants of this type have been performed, and improved survival has been minimal. In the mass casualty radiologic event, most individuals can recover hematopoiesis without a transplant. This type of transplantation may prove to be the only hope for victims with potential stem cell failure, however. Future research in the area of allogenic transplantation is ongoing and may soon represent a more viable treatment option for critically ill patients.

**Summary**

The treatment of injuries from a nuclear weapon or a radioactive dispersal device most likely will be in a mass casualty scenario. Situations with mass casualties are often chaotic, with large numbers of patients and limited resources. Radiation injuries, in combination with burns or mechanical injuries, complicate the treatment process, with increased emphasis on early intervention. Public hysteria in a real or suspected nuclear event may create numerous "worried well" persons [9], who further clog the overwhelmed health care system. These factors suggest that a nuclear event may be the ultimate test of our health care system.

The care of patients must proceed in an orderly fashion, with thoughts toward providing the greatest good to the greatest number. If radiation injury occurs as part of a mass casualty, some organized method of triage, decontamination, evacuation, and treatment must be implemented. Having a system of classification and sorting of radiation-injured casualties, in conjunction with normal procedures of evacuation and hospitalization, decreases the overwhelming demand on the supporting medical facilities.

Oral and maxillofacial surgeons should plan to become integral members of the treatment team, especially considering their wide scope of training. Oral and maxillofacial surgeons can work with the triage team, provide care for head and neck injuries with the surgical team, provide basic overall patient management for the trauma team, and provide assistance for the anesthesia team in a time of need. It is important for all health care providers to become familiar with the types of injuries that can be expected after a radiologic attack and the treatment modalities that can preserve life should such a catastrophe occur.

**Several key points should be restated:**

1. Nuclear threat most likely will be seen as a terrorist attack on a pre-existing nuclear power plant. Other methods of attack could come in the form of nuclear warheads and what have been termed "dirty bombs" or "suitcase bombs."
2. There have been no reports of a health care provider suffering a radiation injury while performing basic life support on an exposed or contaminated patient.
3. Injuries that are most likely to be seen are thermal burns, blast injuries, and penetrating radiation.
4. Time of injury to onset of vomiting is a good predictor for severity of radiation exposure and prognosis.
5. Decontamination of a patient and a patient's wounds requires special considerations as a result of radiation exposure.
6. Surgical therapy should be performed within 36 hours after radiation exposure. Otherwise, surgery should be delayed 6 to 8 weeks.
7. Triage of an injured patient is important while treating mass casualties with varying levels of injuries.
8. Certain medications can be beneficial in the long- and short-term treatment of patients exposed to nuclear radiation.

## References

[1] Willis D, Coleman EA. The dirty bomb: management of victims of radiological weapons. MEDSURG Nursing 2003;12(6):397–401.
[2] United States Nuclear Regulatory Commission. Dirty bombs: fact sheet. Washington (DC): United States Nuclear Regulatory Commission; 2003.
[3] Department of Homeland Security Working Group on Radiological Dispersal Device Preparedness. Medical guidelines for ionizing radiation and terrorist incidents: important points for the patient and you. Washington, DC: US Department of Homeland Security; 2003.
[4] Defense Technical Information Center, United States Army. Damaging factors of nuclear explosions and kinds of injuries caused in man. USAMIIA-K-8070. Washington, DC: Department of the Army; 1977.
[5] Bowen TE, Bellamy R. Mass casualties in thermonuclear warfare. In: Specific medical effects of nuclear weapons: emergency war surgery NATO handbook: Part I. Types of wounds and injuries. Washington, DC: United States Department of Defense; 1988. p. 1–18.
[6] Conklin JJ, Walker RI, Kelleher DL. Evaluation and treatment of nuclear casualties: Part III. Management of combined injuries. Medical Bulletin of the United States Army 1983;40(12):17–21.
[7] Radiological injuries. In: Szul A, editor. Emergency war surgery. Chapter 30. Washington (DC): Library of Congress Cataloging-in-Publication Data, Borden Institute; 2004. p. 30.1–30.7.
[8] Johnston WR. Nuclear weapons effects: an overview. 2004. Available at: http://www.johnstonarchive.net/nuclear/effectsum.html. © 2001–2004, 2005 by Wm. Robert Johnston.
[9] Schleipman AR, Gerbaudo VH, Castronovo FP. Radiation disaster response: preparation and simulation experience at an academic medical center. J Nuclear Medicine Technology 2004;32(1):22–7.

## Further readings

Centers for Disease Control and Prevention. Radiation emergencies: radiation and health effects. Washington, DC: US Department of Health and Human Services. April 7, 2003.

Elcock D, Klemic G, Toboas A. Establishing remediation levels in response to a radiation dispersal event. Environmental Science and Technology 2004;38(9):2505–12.

Internal Peer Review. Maxillofacial wounds and injuries. In: Emergency war surgery NATO handbook: Part IV.

Regional wounds and injuries. Washington, DC: United States Department of Defense; 1988.

Ring JP. Radiation risks and dirty bombs. Health Physics 2004;86(Suppl 1):S42–7.

United States Department of Health and Human Services. Guidance: potassium iodine as a thyroid blocking agent in radiation emergencies. Washington, DC: United States Department of Health and Human Services; 2001.

United States Nuclear Regulatory Commission. Biological effects of radiation: fact sheet. Washington (DC): United States Nuclear Regulatory Commission; 2003.

ELSEVIER
SAUNDERS

Oral Maxillofacial Surg Clin N Am 17 (2005) 299–330

ORAL AND
MAXILLOFACIAL
SURGERY CLINICS
of North America

# Bioterrorism and Biologic Warfare

## Sidney L. Bourgeois, Jr, DDS\*, Michael J. Doherty, DDS

*Department of Oral and Maxillofacial Surgery, National Capital Consortium, National Naval Medical Center,
8901 Wisconsin Avenue, Bethesda, MD 20889, USA*

Biologic warfare has been defined as "the use of micro-organisms or toxins derived from living organisms to produce death or disease in humans, animals, or plants" [1]. Bioterrorism can be defined in the same manner [2]. Although little had been written about bioterrorism in the past, recently the concept of bioterrorism has come to the forefront of the American mind. Many people have dismissed bioterrorism as little more than a theoretical threat. This dismissal has been based on four points of view: (1) Biologic weapons seldom have been used in the past, which suggests that they would not be used. (2) The use of biologic weapons is so morally repugnant that they will not be used. (3) Only the most sophisticated laboratories would be able to produce the agents or contrive a method of dispersal. (4) The potential destructiveness of biologic weapons makes their use unthinkable. These arguments fail to consider the historical precedent of use of biologic weapons [3].

## Historical use of biologic weapons

Two of the earliest recorded uses of a biologic agent in warfare occurred in the sixth century BC. In one event, the Assyrians reportedly poisoned the wells of their enemies with rye ergot, a fungus [4,5]. During the siege of Cirrha in the sixth century, the Athenian politician Solon dumped the herb purgative hellebore into the city's water supply, which resulted in Solon's capture of the city when the troops guarding Cirrha deserted their posts [5]. During a naval battle in 184 BC, the Carthaginians hurled earthen pots filled with "serpents of every kind" onto the decks of Perganum ships. With the Perganum soldiers fighting two enemies, the Carthaginians were victorious [6,7]. In the twelfth century at the Battle of Tortona, Barbarossa contaminated the enemy's wells with the bodies of his dead soldiers in one of the earliest known uses of fomites in an attempt to spread disease [5,8]. Fomites are objects that harbor micro-organisms and can transmit diseases. During the fourteenth-century Tartar siege of Kaffa (currently Feodossia, Ukraine), the attacking Tartar forces experienced an epidemic of plague and catapulted their dead into the city in an attempt to initiate a plague epidemic [7,9]. The "hurling of dead bodies over city walls" also was reportedly used by Russian troops battling Swedish forces in 1710 [7].

Smallpox was used as a biologic weapon on at least three occasions in history. The first occurred when Pizzaro presented variola-contaminated clothing to the indigenous peoples of South America in the fifteenth century. During the French and Indian Wars of 1754 to 1767, the English distributed smallpox-laden blankets to Native American Indians loyal to the French, which resulted in the loss of Fort Carillon and several smallpox outbreaks in various tribes throughout the Ohio Valley [6,7]. During the American Civil War, Confederate surgeon Dr. Luke Blackburn was arrested for importing clothing from

The views expressed in this article are those of the authors and do not necessarily represent the official policy or position of the National Naval Medical Center, the United States Navy, the Department of Defense, or the United States government.

\* Corresponding author.

*E-mail address:* slbourgeois@bethesda.med.navy.mil (S.L. Bourgeois, Jr).

1042-3699/05/\$ – see front matter. Published by Elsevier Inc.
doi:10.1016/j.coms.2005.04.003

patients infected with smallpox and yellow fever and selling them to Union troops [5,10]. During World War I, Germany reportedly shipped horses and cattle inoculated with *Bacillus anthracis* and *Pseudomonas* (currently *Burkholderia*) *pseudomallei* to the United States and other countries. The Germans are also suspected of infecting Romanian sheep that were to be sent to Russia [6,7]. During World War II, the Japanese conducted an ambitious biologic weapons program. The program began in 1932 with numerous human experiments in Manchuria. Unit 731 conducted experiments on prisoners of war using anthrax, botulism, brucellosis, cholera, dysentery, gas gangrene, meningococcal infection, and plague. Participants in the program who were captured by the Soviet Union during the war admitted to 12 large-scale field trials against 11 Chinese cities. Plague allegedly was weaponized by allowing laboratory-bred fleas to feed on plague-infected rats. These potentially infected fleas were then released from aircraft over Chinese cities. The only known German use of biologic warfare was the contamination of a reservoir in northwestern Bohemia with sewage. Hitler reportedly issued orders that prohibited biologic weapons development. The German program was more defensive in nature and revolved around the development of vaccines and antibiotics.

The British experimented with anthrax during World War II on Gruinard Island off the coast of Scotland. These tests contaminated the island until a costly decontamination was completed in 1986. The Viet Cong used feces-contaminated pungi sticks against United States and South Vietnamese forces during the early 1960s [11]. In 1978, the toxin ricin was used to assassinate Georgi Markov, a Bulgarian defector who lived in London, and an attempt was made on Vladimar Kostov's life in Paris [5]. "Iraq has stated that its biological weapons programs dates back to at least 1974." The Iraqi program produced approximately 380,000 L of botulinum toxin, 84,250 L of anthrax spores, 3400 L of *Clostridium perfringens* spores, and 2200 L of aflatoxin. Many weapons were filled with these agents and deployed for action by the end of 1990 [12]. An epidemic of *Salmonella typhimurium* caused 751 cases of gastroenteritis in Oregon in 1984. Although the Centers for Disease Control and Prevention (CDC) linked the source to salad bars in local restaurants, a bioterrorist event was not confirmed until a follower of Bhagwan Shree Rajneesh admitted to the attack. The goal of the attack was to influence a local election [5,11].

The Japanese Aum Shinrikyo cult conducted a sarin nerve gas attack on the Tokyo subway system in March 1995. After an investigation into this chemical attack, previous biologic attacks with anthrax and botulinum toxin were uncovered. Also uncovered during the investigation was a trip to Zaire (currently Democratic Republic of Congo) to collect Ebola virus [5,11,13]. Plans to produce ricin, which were linked to al Qaeda, were found in Kabul, Afghanistan in November 2001. A recipe for ricin production was found on the body of a Chechen rebel in 2003. In London, more than ten individuals were arrested in January 2003 in connection with a potential terrorist plot to use ricin. A South Carolina post office received a package that contained ricin and a threatening note in 2003 [14]. Numerous smaller events were thwarted by law enforcement officials in the United States in the 1980s and 1990s. The Minnesota Patriots Council was preparing to use ricin and the solvent dimethyl sulfoxide to murder federal and local law enforcement agents. The key members were the first people convicted under the Biological Weapons and Antiterrorism Act of 1989. Two teenagers who had created a white supremacist organization dubbed RISE were days away from contaminating the municipal water supply with *S typhimurium* when arrested by the Chicago police in 1982. Another white supremacist, Larry Wayne Harris, was arrested in 1995 for obtaining stocks of *Yersinia pestis*, the bacteria responsible for causing plague, and in 1998 for possession of anthrax and is believed to be responsible for an outbreak of anthrax hoax letters [5]. The most recent instance of bioterrorism involved the anthrax attacks that occurred through the US Postal System in October 2001.

## Biologic weapons proliferation

The first attempt to limit the proliferation and use of biologic weapons occurred after World War I. The 1925 Protocol for the Prohibition of the Use in War of Asphyxiating, Poisonous, or other Gases and of Bacteriological Methods of Warfare—otherwise known as the Geneva Protocol—was the first multilateral agreement to extending prohibition of chemical and biologic agents. Despite this being a landmark event in limiting the production and use of these weapons, the Protocol's effect was virtually inconsequential because there was no provision for verification inspections [7]. Many countries, including the United Kingdom, the former Soviet Union, and France, although signatories, stipulated that they would not be bound to this agreement if their enemies or the allies of their enemies used chemical or biologic weapons. "Thus, the Geneva Protocol became a 'no-first-use' agreement with no legally binding restrictions on the research, development, or deployment of either chemical warfare or biological weapons" [15]. As a result of increasing international concern, Great Britain submitted a proposal to the United Nations Committee on Disarmament in 1969 that prohibited the development, production, and stockpiling of biologic weapons and provided for inspections in response to alleged violations. The following September, the Warsaw Pact nations submitted a similar proposal without the provision for inspections [11]. In 1972, the Convention on the Prohibition of the Development, Production and Stockpiling of Bacteriological and Toxin Weapons and their Destruction, also known as the 1972 Biological Weapons Convention, was developed. The Biological Weapons Convention was signed by 158 nations and ratified by 140 nations and entered into force in 1975 [15]. In 1969 (for micro-organisms) and 1970 (for toxins) President Nixon terminated the United States offensive biologic weapons program and adopted a policy never to use biologic weapons, including toxins, under any circumstance [5,6,11]. Unfortunately, the number of countries known or suspected of having biologic weapons capability has doubled since the Biological Weapons Convention [15]. This fact was substantiated in part by the UN Special Commission on Iraq inspections in Iraq [12], the admission by Boris Yeltsin that the 1979 anthrax outbreak at Sverdlovsk, USSR was the result of an accidental release from a secret biologic warfare facility, and reports from Dr. Kanatjan Alibekov (Ken Alibek), a Soviet defector who was involved with biologic warfare research in the former Soviet Union. He revealed to the United States that the Soviet Union began violating the Biological Weapons Convention soon after signing it [7,11,12,16].

## Potential weapons

The CDC was tasked as part of a Congressional initiative in 1999 to review and comment on the threat potential of various agents using the following information as general criteria: (1) public health impact based on illness and death, (2) delivery potential to large populations based on stability of the agent, ability to mass produce and distribute a virulent agent, and potential for person-to-person transmission of the agent, (3) public perception as related to public fear and potential civil disruption, and (4) special public health preparedness needs based on stockpile requirements, enhanced surveil-

lance, or diagnostic needs. These were classified according to a three-tier system from high-priority agents to emerging threat agents and labeled as Categories A through C [17]. Category A agents are the highest priority agents and include organisms that can be disseminated easily or transmitted person-to-person, cause high mortality, with the potential for major public health impact, have the potential to cause public panic and social disruption, and require special action for public health preparedness. Category B agents are the second highest priority agents and include organisms that are moderately easy to disseminate, cause moderate morbidity and low mortality, and require specific enhancements of CDC diagnostic capacity and enhanced disease surveillance. Category C agents are the third highest priority agents and include emerging pathogens that could be engineered for mass dissemination in the future because of availability; ease of production, and dissemination and have the potential for high morbidity and mortality and major health impact (Table 1) [18].

### Category A agents

#### Smallpox
*History.* A scourge for more than 3000 years, the specter of smallpox is once again upon us. The last naturally occurring case of smallpox occurred in Somalia in 1972. The World Health Organization declared smallpox eradicated in 1980 after an aggressive worldwide immunization program that began in 1967. By 1984, only two laboratories retained variola virus isolates—the CDC in Atlanta and the Research Institute of Viral Preparations in Moscow. In 1994, the Russian isolates were moved to the State Research Center of Virology and Biotechnology (the Vektor Institute) in Novosibirsk, Russia [19]. Questions remain concerning the security of the Russian isolates and of the exportation of equipment and expertise to rogue states.

*Epidemiology.* With the eradication of smallpox, routine vaccination of the public ceased more than 25 years ago. "The deliberate reintroduction of smallpox as an epidemic disease would be a crime of unprecedented proportions." In an unvaccinated, highly susceptible, highly mobile population, second- and third-generation cases would develop rapidly throughout the country and possibly the world, with rates varying between 37% and 88% [19–21]. An outbreak that occurred in Meschede, Germany affected 17 people on three floors secondary to one patient who had a cough and who was not adequately isolated during the incubation period [22]. There is also

Table 1
Centers for Disease Control and Prevention critical biologic agent categories

| Biologic agents | Disease |
| --- | --- |
| **Category A** | |
| Variola major | Smallpox |
| B anthracis | Anthrax |
| Y pestis | Plague |
| Clostridium botulinum (botulinum toxins) | Botulism |
| Francisella tularensis | Tularemia |
| Filovirus (Marburg and Ebola) | Viral hemorrhagic fevers |
| Arenavirus (Lassa, Argentine/Junin) | Viral hemorrhagic fevers |
| | |
| **Category B** | |
| Coxiella burnetii | Q fever |
| Brucella spp. | Brucellosis |
| Burkholderia mallei | Glanders |
| B pseudomallei | Melioidosis |
| Alphaviruses (VEE, EEE, WEE) | Encephalitis |
| Rickettsia prowaekii | Typhus fever |
| Toxins[a] | Toxic syndromes |
| Chlamydia psittaci | Psittacosis |
| Food safety threats (Salmonella spp., E. coli O157:H7) | |
| Water threats (Vibrio cholera, Cryptosporidium parvum) | |
| | |
| **Category C** | |
| Emerging pathogens[b] | |

Abbreviations: EEE, Eastern equine encephalitis; VEE, Venezuelan equine encephalitis; WEE, Western equine encephalitis.
   [a] Ricin, staphylococcal enterotoxin B, epsilon toxin — C perfringens.
   [b] Nipah virus, Hantavirus, tickborne encephalitis virus, tickborne hemorrhagic fever virus, yellow fever, multidrug-resistant tuberculosis.
Data from CDC Strategic Planning Workgroup. Biological and chemical terrorism: strategic plan for preparedness and response. Recommendations of the CDC strategic planning workgroup. MMWR Morb Mortal Wkly Rep 2000;49(No. RR-4):1–14.

increased concern regarding patients with immunodeficiencies or medically induced immunosuppression. The discovery of a single suspected case of smallpox must be treated as an international health emergency, and local, state, and federal health authorities must be notified. There are two principle forms and three rare forms of the disease: (1) variola major, which accounted for approximately 90% of the cases, with case fatality rates of approximately 30% in unvaccinated persons and approximately 3% in vaccinated persons; (2) variola minor (alastrim), a much milder form that accounted for 2% of cases and had a case fatality rate of ≤1%; (3) the flat or malignant type, which accounted for 7% of cases and had a case fatality rate of 97% in unvaccinated people; (4) the hemorrhagic type, which accounted for fewer than 3% of cases and was uniformly fatal; (5) variola sine eruptione, which occurred in previously vaccinated contacts or in infants with maternal antibodies, was not fatal, produced no rash, and lasted less the 48 hours [19,20,23]. Humans are the only known reservoir of variola major; no animal

or insect reservoir has ever been identified. Although monkeypox, vaccinia, and cowpox can infect humans, only smallpox is readily transmitted from person to person [24]. There is a seasonal variation, with the historical incidence being highest during the winter and early spring, which correlates with the higher survivability of the virus at lower temperatures and low humidity [19,20,25,26].

Microbiology.    Smallpox is caused by the variola virus, a DNA virus of the genus Orthopoxvirus. The Orthopoxvirus family also includes vaccinia, monkeypox virus, cowpox, and others [24]. All Orthopoxvirus genomes are similar to each other [27]. The virion is characteristically brick-shaped and has a diameter of 200 nm.

Pathogenesis and clinical presentation.    Smallpox spreads primarily by droplets or aerosols from the oropharynx of infected people but also can be spread by fomites. Infection occurs after implantation of the virus on oropharyngeal or respiratory mucosa [20].

The viral particles migrate rapidly into local lymph nodes and multiply. The infectious dose is believed to be only a few virions [22]. A brief asymptomatic viremia occurs on or about the third or fourth day. The viremia is followed by a latent period of 4 to 14 days, during which virus multiplication occurs in the reticuloendothelial system. A second viremia occurs and precedes the prodrome phase. During this second viremia the virus invades the capillary epithelium of the dermal layer of the skin and beneath the oropharyngeal mucosa. At the end of the incubation period, 7 to 17 days (mean, 10–12 days), the patient enters the prodrome phase, which is characterized by the abrupt onset of high fever (>40°C), headache, backache, and malaise and, occasionally, severe abdominal pain and delirium. This prodrome phase typically subsides in 2 to 3 days. An enanthema then arises over the tongue and oropharynx and precedes the maculopapular rash by a day. The rash begins as small, reddish macules and becomes papular with a diameter of 2 to 3 mm over 1 to 2 days. Within another 2 days the papules become vesicular and have a diameter of 2 to 5 mm. The lesions begin on the face and extremities, including the palms and soles, before the trunk. A defining characteristic is that all lesions are in the same stage of development. Four to seven days after the onset of the rash, the vesicles become pustular. The pustules are round, tense, and deeply embedded in the dermis. Crusts begin to form between the eighth and ninth day of the rash.

As patients recover, the scabs separate to reveal the characteristic pock marks or pitted scarring, which occurs in 65% to 80% of survivors. The characteristic scars are most evident on the face secondary to destruction of sebaceous glands followed by shrinking of granulation tissue and fibrosis [19,20]. A list of otologic, nasal, and ocular complications of smallpox can be found in Box 1 [28,29]. Encephalitis occasionally occurs. Death usually occurs during the second week of the disease, likely secondary to toxemia. The flat or malignant type is characterized by abrupt onset and prostrating constitutional symptoms. The confluent lesions evolve slowly and never progress to the pustular stage but remain soft, flattened, and velvety to the touch. The skin has the appearance of a fine-grained, reddish-colored crepe rubber. If a patient survives, the lesions gradually disappear without forming scabs; large amounts of epidermis sometimes slough off. The hemorrhagic type occurs among all ages and in both sexes, but pregnant women seem to be unusually susceptible. Illness usually begins with a shorter incubation period and a severely prostrating prodromal illness. Soon, a

> **Box 1. Otologic, nasal, and ocular complications of smallpox**
>
> Acute necrotizing otitis media
> Conductive hearing loss
> Sensorineural hearing loss
> Necrosis of the turbinates
> Epistaxis
> Nasal vestibular stenosis secondary to internal and external nasal scarring
> Panophthalmitis
> Blindness
> Iritis
> Iridocyclitis
> Secondary glaucoma
> Paralysis of extraocular muscles
> Retrobulbar hemorrhage
> Disciform keratitis
> Ankyloblepharon
> Ectropion
> Obstruction of the lacrimal punctum
> Orbital cellulitis
> Choroiditis
> Dacryocystitis
> Optic neuritis
> Optic atrophy
>
> *Data from* Tennyson HC, Mair EA. Smallpox: what every otolaryngologist should know. Otolaryngol Head Neck Surg 2004; 130(3):323–33; Semba RD. The ocular complications of smallpox and smallpox immunization. Arch Ophthalmol 2003; 121(5):715–9.

dusky erythema develops, which is followed by petechiae and frank hemorrhages into the skin and mucous membranes. The altered clinical appearance of the flat and hemorrhagic type seems to be related to a local inhibition of cell-mediated immunity [30]. Death usually occurs by the fifth or sixth day after onset of the rash. Variola minor has a less severe course, with fewer constitutional symptoms and a more limited rash [20]. People with smallpox are considered infectious from the appearance of the rash until the last scab falls off.

*Diagnosis.* Diagnosis depends on recognizing clinical features and laboratory confirmation. A recently vaccinated person (or one who was vaccinated that day) who is wearing personal protective equipment and observing airborne and contact precautions should collect the specimen. Vesicular or pustular lesions are opened with the blunt edge of a scalpel, and the fluid is harvested on a sterile cotton swab. Scabs also can be used and can be picked off with forceps. Specimens are deposited in a vacutainer tube. The junction of the stopper and tube is sealed with adhesive tape. The entire tube should be secured in a durable, watertight container. Local and state laboratories should be contacted immediately regarding the shipping of specimens. Examination of the specimen requires high-containment (biosafety level 4) facilities, such as at the CDC or the US Army Medical Research Institute of Infectious Diseases (USAMRIID). Confirmation of smallpox can be made by demonstrating the presence of virions by electron microscopy, demonstrating viral antigen by immunohistochemical studies, identifying variola virus by polymerase chain reaction (PCR) assay for orthopoxvirus genes and isolation of the virus on livecell cultures, and using nucleic acid identification of *Orthopoxvirus* species or growth on chorioallantois [19].

Diseases that should be considered in a differential diagnosis are other poxviruses, measles, varicella/chickenpox, herpes zoster, drug eruptions, erythema multiforme, molluscum contagiosum, scabies, secondary syphilis, insect bites, and vesiculobullous disorders [24]. Varicella is one diagnosis that causes the most confusion with smallpox. There are several defining characteristics that separate the two, however. First, all smallpox lesions develop at the same pace, and on any part of the body the lesions appear identical. Conversely, chickenpox lesions develop at different rates, and on any part of the body lesions in several different stages of development are present. Second, smallpox lesions have a predilection for the face and extremities, including the palms and soles, whereas chickenpox lesions are denser on the trunk and are almost never seen on the palms or soles. The pustules of smallpox also have a central umbilication (belly button–like) [30], whereas the pustules of chickenpox are described as "dew drops on a rose petal." A risk algorithm tool on the CDC's Website can help evaluate a suspicious rash for smallpox (www.bt.cdc.gov/agent/smallpox/diagnosis/riskalgorithm/index.asp).

*Treatment.* No treatment for smallpox has been approved by the US Food and Drug Administration. If lesions become secondarily infected, a penicillinase-resistant antibiotic should be used. Supportive measures are the mainstays of treatment. If a patient is diagnosed within 3 days of exposure to the virus, he or she should be vaccinated. Vaccination within this time frame may prevent disease or decrease the severity of disease and risk of death. The smallpox vaccine is a live virus vaccine made from vaccinia virus (another *Orthopoxvirus*) [31]. No evidence exists that the use of vaccinia immunoglobulin given early in the incubation period along with vaccination provides any additional survival benefit [24]. There is no benefit to using vaccinia immunoglobulin in patients with clinical smallpox [19]. Animal studies demonstrated that cidofovir is active against various orthopoxviruses if given within 1 to 2 days of exposure. The drug could be made available through an investigational new drug protocol in the event of an outbreak [19,20]. Topical antiviral agents, such as idoxuridine, trifluridine, and vidarabine, have been used to treat vaccinia of the cornea and conjunctiva or prevent corneal or conjunctival involvement in patients with eyelid lesions secondary to complications of vaccination [29]. Although their efficacy is unproven for the treatment of ocular complications of smallpox, these medications should be considered for ocular lesions associated with smallpox [19].

*Infection Control and Prevention.* Early diagnosis with proper infection control, isolation, and prevention with an aggressive vaccination program for priority groups are the cornerstones of preventing a pandemic [21]. As soon as the diagnosis of smallpox is made, all individuals in whom smallpox is suspected should be isolated, and all face-to-face or household contacts should be vaccinated and placed under surveillance. The Working Group on Civilian Biodefense recommended that patients be isolated in the home or other nonhospital facility when possible secondary to the threat to hospitals by aerosol dissemination [20,22]. If patients are admitted to the hospital, it is recommended that they be placed in negative-pressure isolation rooms with high-efficiency particulate arresting filtration systems. All personnel who have contact with affected patients should be vaccinated and use airborne and contact precautions in addition to standard universal precautions. All contaminated materials (ie, laundry and waste) should be placed in biohazard bags and should be autoclaved before incineration or washing. Standard hospital-grade disinfecting solutions can be used to clean fixed surfaces [20,32,33].

People who survive an infection retain lifelong immunity. Historically, the first vaccination attempts seem to be made by the Chinese, who created a powder out of the scabs of a patient who survived a mild form of smallpox and instilled the powder into the vaccinee's nose to prevent an infection. In other areas, notably India and Europe, the contents of a lesion were inserted into a cut in the skin [21], a process called variolation. The modern era of vaccination is attributed to Edward Jenner. He observed that milkmaids who were frequently exposed to cowpox seemed never to contract smallpox. He performed extensive research and experimentation with cowpox as a method of providing protection from smallpox. Ultimately, in 1796, Jenner introduced material from a milkmaid's cowpox lesions into the arm of an 8-year-old boy. When subsequently challenged with smallpox, the boy did not contract the disease. He called this use of cowpox to provide protection from smallpox "vaccination," *vacca* being the Latin word for cow.

The current vaccine is a lyophilized formulation of the New York City Board of Health strain of vaccinia virus, which has been used for decades. The vaccine is prepared from the lymph of calves inoculated with vaccinia virus [34]. There are current questions about the immunity level of people vaccinated before smallpox eradication. More than 95% of successful primarily immunized people retain full immunity for 5 to 10 years; successful revaccination provides protection for 10 to 20 years or more [24]. Vaccination initiates a local immune response that results in a combined cellular and humoral immune response [30]. The following contraindications to vaccine administration should be noted: (1) pregnancy or living with someone who is pregnant, (2) immunodeficiencies, (3) extensive skin diseases, such as burns, wounds, recent incisions, impetigo, contact dermatitis, (4) immunosuppressive therapies, (5) inflammatory eye diseases, (6) atopic dermatitis or eczema, whether present, past, or healed, (7) allergy to vaccine component, (8) breastfeeding, and (9) children younger than 12 months of age. The vaccine is administered as noted in Box 2 [35]. After 3 to 5 days in primary vaccinations, a papule forms at the vaccination site. The papule then becomes vesicular (Jennerian vesicle) and progresses to a pustule at approximately day 8. The pustule scabs over between 10 and 14 days. The scab falls off between 17 and 21 days. This progression from papule to pustule signifies a "take" and the development of an immune response [34].

Minor local reactions to the vaccine include formation of satellite lesions, lymphadenopathy, lymphangitis, erythema, edema, pain, pruritis, fever, malaise, nausea, myalgias, and headache. Occasionally a "robust take" occurs, with the surrounding local reaction becoming ≥10 cm in diameter. The robust take usually manifests itself between 8 and 10 days after vaccination and generally improves in 1 to 3 days. Secondary bacterial infections can occur

---

**Box 2. Step-by-step instructions for the administration of smallpox vaccine**

1. Review patient history for contra-indications.

2. Choose the site for vaccination. The deltoid area on the upper arm is recommended.

3. No skin preparation is required. Do not use alcohol preparation before vaccination because it has been shown to inactivate the virus.

4. Dip the bifurcated needle into the vial of vaccine (0.0025 mL of vaccine is held between the tines of the needle) [35]. The same needle never should be dipped into the vaccine vial more than once to prevent contamination of the vial.

5. Insert the needle perpendicularly to the skin within a 5-mm diameter area. The needle is inserted 3 times for primary vaccination and 15 times for revaccination. A trace of blood should appear at the vaccination site within 15 to 20 seconds. If no trace of blood is visible, an additional 3 insertions of the needle are performed. The needle is for one-time use only.

6. Absorb excess vaccine with sterile gauze and discard the gauze in an appropriate biohazardous waste receptacle.

7. Cover the vaccination site.
   a. Secure gauze loosely by first-aid adhesive tape.
   b. If working in a health care setting, keep the vaccination site covered with a semipermeable dressing over the gauze.

8. Educate the vaccinee or guardian or both.
   a. Do not rub or scratch the vaccination site.
   b. Keep the site covered and change gauze-only dressings every 1 to 2 days or if wet and semipermeable dressings every 3 to 5 days.
   c. Discard the dressing in plastic zip bags.
   d. Set aside a laundry hamper for linen items that may come into contact with the vaccination site.
   e. Wash all linen materials that come into contact with the vacci-

nation site in hot water with detergent or bleach or both.
  f. Wash hands after touching vacci-
     nation site or objects that come
     into contact with vaccination site.
  g. When the scab falls off, throw it
     away in a plastic zip bag.
  h. Report any problems to the per-
     son or organization noted on the
     post-vaccination and follow-up
     information sheet, a health care
     provider, or health care personnel
     at an emergency room.
  i. Return to the immunizing provider
     to check for a positive "take."
9. Record the vaccination.

*From* Lane JM, Ruben FL, Neff JM, Millar
JD. Complications of smallpox vaccination, 1968: results of 10 statewide surveys. J Infect Dis 1970;122(4):303–9;
with permission.

within 5 days of vaccination or beyond 30 days and continue to progress if not treated with antibiotics [36]. The information on adverse reactions has been based on ten statewide surveys in 1968. Adverse reactions include (1) erythema multiforme, (2) accidental inoculation, (3) generalized vaccinia, (4) eczema vaccinatum, (5) progressive vaccinia, (6) post-vaccination encephalitis, and (7) myocarditis [20,30, 34,37]. The availability of vaccinia immunoglobulin is limited. Researchers recommend that its use should be reserved for the most serious cases [20]. Vaccinia immunoglobulin is indicated for the treatment of eczema vaccinatum, progressive vaccinia, extensive accidental inoculation, and severe or recurrent generalized vaccinia [34,36]. The CDC recommends that varicella vaccination and purified protein derivative tests not be administered within 4 weeks of vaccinia. The delay is recommended so as not to confuse potential vaccine reactions and not alter the purified protein derivative results [35].

*Smallpox as a Weapon.* There is conclusive evidence of the production of large quantities of weaponized smallpox by the former Soviet Union. Soviet experts concluded that smallpox as a weapon was incomparable based on the following factors: (1) its infectious dose with and lethal dose (LD)50 of only 10 to 20 viral particles, (2) its stability in an aerosol, (3) its ability to travel for many miles without

the loss of virulence, (4) its ability to survive in the environment, (5) the number of susceptible personnel secondary to a halt of vaccinations, and (6) its highly contagious state. A modern biologic attack could occur in several ways: (1) through contamination of articles and food, 2) through use of mechanical devices to generate an aerosol, (3) through use of an explosive device, (4) through use of "natural" air movements (eg, subway, elevators) to generate an aerosol [38], and (5) through use of an intentionally infected "suicide" terrorist to spread the disease [38,39].

*Post-event sequelae.* There will be a need for mental health management during and after a bioterrorist event [40]. Should the need arise to take infected patients to the operating room, the hospital should have an operating room policy on treating patients infected with smallpox. Some adjustments may need to be made on the part of oral and maxillofacial surgeons to treat acutely injured patients if treatment is required on an emergent basis, including, but not limited to, vaccination, removal of unnecessary supplies and equipment from the operating room, wearing of N-95 particulate respirator-type masks, and following the transportation and decontamination route according to hospital policy [41]. Patients who survive may be horribly disfigured and have pockmarks on the face. Historically, these have been treated with dermabrasion with considerable success [42,43].

*Anthrax*
*History.* The earliest references to anthrax are found in the book of Exodus, which describes the fifth and sixth plagues of Egypt in 1491 BC. The best ancient description is by the Roman poet Virgil (70–19 BC) [44]. The disease became known as "the Black Bane" in the Middle Ages [45]. Anthrax was the prototype for Koch's Postulates on disease transmission. Pasteur used the first vaccine that contained attenuated live organisms of *Bacillus anthracis* [44]. The term "anthrax" derives from the Greek word *anthrakis*, which means coal, because the cutaneous form displays black, coal-like lesions. John Bell recognized *B anthracis* as the cause of woolsorter's disease (inhalational anthrax) [45].

*Epidemiology.* Anthrax is a worldwide zoonosis that most commonly occurs in herbivores (eg, cattle, horses, sheep, and goats). Human cases are invariably zoonotic in origin; however, the Sverdlovsk incident and the events of September and October 2001 changed that. Historically, human cases were secondary to contact with infected animals or animal products [45]. In April 1979, at least 66 human deaths occurred in a 4-km path downwind from a biologic weapons plant in Sverdlovsk, USSR. Livestock involved in the incident died as far away as 50 km [46]. Cases of anthrax in the United States were almost unheard of before the terrorist attacks in 2001. From 1978 to 1998, there was less than 1 case of anthrax per year reported in the United States [45]. Human anthrax occurs in three major forms: (1) inhalational, (2) cutaneous, and (3) gastrointestinal. Gastrointestinal anthrax exhibits two subtypes, oropharyngeal and abdominal [47].

*Microbiology.* *B anthracis* is an aerobic, grampositive, spore-forming, nonmotile bacteria. Anthrax spores can survive in their dormant state for decades before they come into contact with a host through breaks in the skin, inhalation, or ingestion. The British experience on Gruinard Island bears this out, because the spores remained viable for 36 years until decontamination began in 1979. Spores are resistant to drying, heating, ultraviolet light, gamma radiation, and many disinfectants. Spores are induced to germinate into their vegetative form when they contact an environment that is rich in nutrients, has a temperature of at least 37°C, and has a carbon dioxide level of at least 5%. Once nutrients are exhausted or the environment becomes unfavorable (eg, pH <6, drought, increased rainfall), sporulation occurs [48,49]. On Gram stain, the spores appear as central unstained areas. In vitro, the bacteria frequently occur in long chains, which gives them a jointed bamboo rod appearance. In vivo, the bacteria appear as individual organisms or at most in chains of two to three organisms [50]. An India ink or polychrome methylene blue stain may allow for better visualization of the capsule [50,51].

The virulence of *B anthracis* requires a three-component protein exotoxin and a poly-D-glutamic acid capsule encoded by plasmids pX01 and pX02, respectively. The capsule is weakly antigenic and antiphagocytic. Strains with a pX02 deletion and no capsule are avidly phagocytosed by leukocytes [45,48,52]. The first component of the exotoxin is called Protective Antigen because it is the main protective constituent of anthrax vaccine. The second component is Edema Factor, a calmodulin-dependent adenyl cyclase. The third component is Lethal Factor, a protease that cleaves mitogen-activated protein kinases 1 and 2. Protective Antigen binds to a target cell surface receptor, and a segment of the protein is cleaved, which exposes a second binding site and allows binding with Edema Factor to form edema toxin or with Lethal Factor to form lethal Toxin

[45,48,52]. The toxins are transported across the cell membrane; the factors are released into the cytosol, where they exert their effects. Edema Factor acts by converting ATP to cyclic AMP, which increases intracellular cyclic AMP levels and leads to edema. The action of lethal factor is less well understood but is believed to be a metalloproteinase with the ability to lyse macrophages while inducing the release of tumor necrosis factor and interleukin 1 [45].

Cutaneous anthrax is the most common form and accounts for 90% to 95% of worldwide cases. This form develops after the introduction of spores into the subcutaneous tissues through cuts or abrasions, which occurs primarily on exposed skin, such as the face, neck, and extremities [52]. Although scarring is minimal [51], eyelid involvement can lead to cicatrization and ectropion [53–55]. Facial palsy also has been reported after cutaneous anthrax [55]. Patients may develop dyspnea and airway compromise [52]. At the site of introduction of spores into the subcutaneous tissue, a papule develops after an incubation period of 12 hours to 19 days, with an average of 2 to 3 days. Within 1 to 2 days, the papule ulcerates, enlarges, and manifests accompanying vesicles [48,51,52]. Regional lymphadenopathy may occur [48,51]. The ulcer progresses into a depressed, painless, black eschar that dries and falls off in 1 to 2 weeks [48,51,52]. Fever is rarely present.

Gastrointestinal anthrax accounts for approximately 2.5% to 5% of cases. Some researchers classify oropharyngeal anthrax as a separate entity [50], whereas others classify it as a subtype of gastrointestinal anthrax along with the abdominal subtype [51]. Some controversy exists over whether gastrointestinal anthrax occurs because of ingestion of spores or the vegetative form in poorly cooked meat. Few countries outside of Africa and Asia have reported cases of gastrointestinal anthrax. In the abdominal subtype, initial symptoms are nausea, vomiting, anorexia, and fever. With disease progression, severe abdominal pain that resembles an acute abdomen occurs. Pain is followed by hematemesis, bloody diarrhea, septicemia, and, ultimately, death. The characteristic eschar occurs most often on the wall of the terminal ileum or cecum. The symptoms result from severe and widespread necrosis of the initial eschar together with extreme edema of the mesentery and intestines and enlargement of local mesenteric lymph nodes [51]. The oropharyngeal subtype is generally considered to be caused by spores lodging in the oropharynx and resulting in anthrax-like nodules or ulcers on the tonsils, pharynx, or hard palate [56]. Sore throat, dysphagia, fever, cervical lymphadenopathy, edema, and airway compromise may be seen [57,58]. The ulcers may be covered with a gray pseudomembrane that resembles diphtheria [52].

Inhalational anthrax accounts for approximately 2.5% to 5% of sporadic cases. The dissemination of spores via an aerosol and subsequent infection are linked to spore size. Spores larger than 5 μm cannot affect the lungs because they are either trapped in the nasopharynx or cleared by mucociliary action. Spore sizes between 2 and 5 μm can lodge in the alveoli, where the disease process begins. Once in the alveoli, the spores are phagocytosed by macrophages and are transported to mediastinal and hilar lymph nodes. After a period of germination, a large amount of toxin is produced, which overwhelms regional lymph nodes. The toxin finds its way into the systemic circulation and results in edema, necrosis, hemorrhage, sepsis, and death. Hemorrhagic mediastinitis is typical of inhalational anthrax [46]. The LD50 for humans is extrapolated from animal data and is estimated to be 2500 to 55,000 spores. Recent primate data suggest that as few as 1 to 3 spores may be sufficient to cause infection [47]. Inhalational anthrax is not a true pneumonia because the bronchoalveolar lung tissue is not primarily affected [56]. The disease course is typically biphasic. The onset of symptoms in the 2001 attacks began 4 to 6 days after inhalation of spores, whereas in Sverdlovsk, the onset of symptoms began 2 to 43 days after inhalation [59]. The initial stage begins insidiously with the onset of "flu-like" symptoms of myalgia, malaise, fatigue, nonproductive cough, retrosternal pressure, and fever and lasts an average of 4 days. Symptoms may improve slightly before the second stage. In the second stage of infection, the patient develops acute respiratory distress, pleural effusions, hypoxemia, and cyanosis that may rapidly culminate in death. The pleural effusions are often massive and hemorrhagic in nature [59].

Anthrax meningitis can occur via hematogenous spread from mediastinal or hilar lymph nodes [59], which occurs as an end-stage process of any form of anthrax [51]. The clinical signs are similar to those of any bacterial meningitis, fever, fatigue, myalgia, nausea, vomiting, seizures, agitation, nuchal rigidity, and delirium [51,52]. Hemorrhagic meningitis should raise the suspicion of an anthrax infection. Rapid neurologic decline occurs; death follows rapidly 1 to 6 days after onset of symptoms [48].

*Diagnosis.* Successful diagnosis requires a high level of suspicion. The most useful microbiologic test is the standard blood culture, which should show growth in 6 to 24 hours. Cultures should be drawn before the initiation of antibiotic therapy [47]. Correct interpretation of culture results is also vitally important because sometimes a gram-positive bacillus may be dismissed as a contaminant [60,61]. If cutaneous anthrax is suspected, culture and Gram stain of vesicular fluid should be performed. If the results of the Gram stain and cultures are negative and a diagnosis of anthrax is still being entertained, a punch biopsy from the center of the eschar and the surrounding erythematous area should be performed [56]. The specimen should be sent to the CDC laboratory in Atlanta, Georgia or the USAMRIID at Fort Detrick, Maryland. These laboratories have the ability to perform immunohistochemical staining, PCR assays, and enzyme-linked immunosorbent assays (ELISA) for determination of antibodies to Protective Antigen [62]. Sputum Gram stain and cultures are of little value with an absence of a pneumonic process. The CDC has recommended that nasal swabs not be used as a clinical diagnostic test. The nasal swab test may be used for epidemiologic purposes only. If the results of the nasal swab are positive, however, the patient should receive post-exposure antibiotics. (See the section on treatment regimens.) Negative results on a nasal swab should not be used to rule out an anthrax infection or exposure [47]. Inhalational anthrax can be diagnosed using a chest radiograph. A widened mediastinum on a chest radiograph in an otherwise healthy individual with "flu-like" symptoms is considered pathognomonic for inhalational anthrax by some providers [52,62]. Others believe that mediastinal widening is a nonspecific finding because it also can be seen in other conditions, such as tuberculosis, sarcoidosis, histoplasmosis, lymphoma, tumors, and aneurysm [59]. CT of the chest is a diagnostically important study and was abnormal in all patients in which it was performed. CT revealed characteristic abnormalities, such as pleural effusions, perihilar infiltrates, and mediastinal edema. Of significant help in differentiating inhalational anthrax from viral illnesses is the absence of sore throat and rhinorrhea in inhalational anthrax.

The differential diagnosis of cutaneous anthrax includes (1) brown recluse spider bite, (2) ecthyma/impetigo, (3) rat bite fever, (4) plague, (5) typhus, (6) glanders, (7) rickettsial pox, (8) mucormycosis, (9) aspergillosis, (10) cutaneous leishmaniasis, (11) ulceroglandular tularemia, (12) accidental vaccinia, and (13) necrotic herpes simplex. The differential diagnosis of oropharyngeal anthrax includes (1) peritonsillar abscess, (2) parapharyngeal space abscess, (3) streptococcal pharyngitis, (4) Ludwig's angina, and (5) diphtheria. If anthrax meningitis is suspected, lumbar puncture is recommended. Cerebrospinal fluid (CSF) reveals a polymorphonuclear neutrophil predominance with abundant red blood cells. The CSF glucose is depressed, and CSF protein is variably elevated. CSF Gram stain shows gram-positive bacilli. Autopsy results from the Sverdlovsk incident showed a diffuse hemorrhage over the brain that involved the leptomeninges; the condition was called "the Cardinal's Cap" [63].

*Treatment.* Mortality in untreated cases of cutaneous anthrax is estimated at 5% to 20%. Treated cutaneous anthrax has a mortality rate of <1%. Antibiotics are advocated early, but they have no effect on symptoms produced by toxin production [56]. Historically, almost all naturally occurring strains have been susceptible to penicillin, which was the drug of choice. Table 2 provides specific antibiotic recommendations [64–66]. Débridement of the eschar is contraindicated and may increase the likelihood of a secondary bacteremia and scarring [48,67–70]. This is somewhat controversial, because some researchers believe that punch biopsies qualify as incision and débridement and others do not [67]. There are reports of cutaneous débridement of the eschar and treatment with skin grafting [71]. Gastrointestinal anthrax mortality rates are not precisely known but are estimated to be from 4% to 50% [71]. Table 3 provides specific

antibiotic treatment [64–66,72]. Inhalational mortality rates historically have been high (>85%). In the 2001 bioterrorist event, a 40% mortality rate was noted. This improvement in survival is attributed to multidrug antibiotic regimens and advances in modern critical care medicine [73]. Patients may require mechanical ventilation, tube thoracostomy, and other critical care interventions [74]. In animal experiments, antibiotic therapy has prevented development of an immune response. The Working Group recommends continuing antibiotic therapy for 60 days in survivors to prevent recurrence of disease because of the possibility of delayed germination of spores [47]. For cases of anthrax meningitis, steroids may be considered valuable along with the use of an antibiotic with good CNS penetration. Survivors of the recent attacks were treated with a combination of ciprofloxacin and rifampin (for increased gram-positive coverage and its intracellular mechanism of action) and clindamycin (for its ability to prevent expression of toxin) [50,56].

*Infection control and prevention.* Ciprofloxacin, doxycycline, and penicillin G procaine are approved by the US Food and Drug Administration for postexposure prophylaxis of inhalational anthrax [72]. Postexposure prophylaxis for 60 days has been shown to have a poor compliance percentage

Table 2
Recommended therapy for cutaneous anthrax

| Category | Initial therapy[a,d] | Duration of therapy |
|---|---|---|
| Adult and pregnant women[b] | Ciprofloxacin, 500 mg orally twice a day or Doxycycline, 100 mg orally twice a day | 60 d |
| Children[c] <2 y | Ciprofloxacin, 10 mg/kg IV twice a day (maximum dose, 400 mg) or Doxycycline, 2.2 mg/kg IV twice a day (maximum dose, 100 mg) | 60 d |
| Children[c] >2 y | Ciprofloxacin, 15 mg/kg orally twice a day (maximum 1g/d) or Doxycycline, 2.2 mg/kg orally twice a day (maximum dose, 100 mg) | 60 d |

[a] Immunocompromised patients are dosed as per the recommendations for nonimmunocompromised adults and children.

[b] As soon as susceptibilities demonstrate sensitivity to penicillin, pregnant women should be switched to amoxicillin, 500 mg three times a day.

[c] As soon as susceptibilities demonstrate sensitivity to penicillin, children should be switched to amoxicillin, 80 mg/kg three times a day, not to exceed 500 mg/dose.

[d] *B anthracis* exhibits natural resistance to sulfamethoxazole/trimethoprim, cefuroxime, cefotaxime, aztreonam, and ceftazadime. They are not recommended for use [47]. Amoxicillin also may be used for completion of 60-day antibiotic course in children or pregnant or breastfeeding women with cutaneous or inhalational anthrax whose clinical illness has resolved after treatment with primary regimen (14–21 days for inhalational or complicated cutaneous anthrax and 7–10 days for uncomplicated cutaneous anthrax) [72].

*Data from* Centers for Disease Control and Prevention. Update: investigation of anthrax associated with intentional exposure and interim public health guidelines, October 2001. MMWR Morb Mortal Wkly Rep 2001;50(41):890–908; Centers for Disease Control and Prevention. Update: interim recommendations for antimicrobial prophylaxis for children and breastfeeding mothers and treatment of children with anthrax. MMWR Morb Mortal Wkly Rep 2001;50(45):1014–6.

Table 3
Recommended therapy for inhalational and gastrointestinal anthrax[a]

| Category | Contained setting | Duration of therapy | Mass casualty setting | Alternative (If susceptible) | Duration of therapy |
|---|---|---|---|---|---|
| Adult | Ciprofloxacin, 400 mg IV twice a day or Doxycycline, 100 mg IV twice a day and 1–2 additional antimicrobials[b] Switch to oral medications when clinically appropriate Ciprofloxacin, 500 mg orally twice a day or Doxycycline, 100 mg orally twice a day | 60 d | Ciprofloxacin, 500 mg orally twice a day | Doxycycline, 100 mg orally twice a day or Amoxicillin, 500 mg orally three times a day | 60 d |
| Children | Ciprofloxacin, 10 mg/kg IV twice a day (maximum dose, 400 mg) or Doxycycline, 2.2 mg/kg IV twice a day (maximum dose, 100 mg) and 1–2 additional antimicrobials[b] Switch to oral medications when clinically appropriate Ciprofloxacin, 15 mg/kg orally twice a day (maximum 1 g/d) | 60 d | Ciprofloxacin, 15 mg/kg orally twice a day (maximum 1 g/d) | Amoxicillin, 80 mg/kg orally three times a day (maximum dose, 500 mg three times a day) | 60 d |
| Pregnant women | Same as for nonpregnant adult | 60 d | Ciprofloxacin, 500 mg orally twice a day | Amoxicillin, 500 mg orally three times a day | 60 d |

[a] Immunocompromised patients are dosed as per the recommendations for non-immunocompromised adults and children.
[b] Other agents with in vitro activity are rifampin, vancomycin, penicillin, ampicillin, chloramphenicol, imipenem, clindamycin, and clarithromycin.
*Data from* Centers for Disease Control and Prevention. Update: investigation of anthrax associated with international exposure and interim public health guidelines, October 2001. MMWR Morb Mortal Wkly Rep 2001;50(41):890–908; Centers for Disease Control and Prevention. Update: interim recommendations for antimicrobial prophylaxis for children and breastfeeding mothers and treatment of children with anthrax. MMWR Morb Mortal Wkly Rep 2001;50(45):1014–6.

(approximately 42% in the 2001 attacks). In an effort to potentially shorten the duration of postexposure antibiotic treatment to 30 days, a patient may elect to have the anthrax vaccine administered at 0, 2, and 4 weeks [75–77]. The CDC currently only recommends pre-exposure vaccination for people at risk for repeated exposure (eg, military personnel, laboratory workers, and veterinarians) [77]. The anthrax vaccine adsorbed is the only licensed vaccine in the United States. All three toxin components (Lethal Factor, Edema Factor, Protective Antigen) are present in the vaccine. The dosing schedule is not well defined but consists of subcutaneous injections at 0, 2, 4 weeks and 6, 12, 18 months, with an annual booster. The

duration of efficacy of anthrax vaccine adsorbed in humans is unknown. Contraindications to vaccination include previous history of anthrax infection and anaphylactic reaction to a previous dose of anthrax vaccine adsorbed or any of the vaccine components. Adverse reactions to the vaccine have included erythema, mild to severe edema, fever, myalgias, nausea, arthralgia, headache, asthenia, pruritis, anaphylaxis, cellulitis, pneumonia, Guillain-Barré syndrome, seizures, cardiomyopathy, systemic lupus erythematosus, multiple sclerosis, collagen vascular disease, sepsis, angioedema, and transverse myelitis [76,77]. Human-to-human transmission seems not to occur or is exceedingly rare [33,48,74]. Standard universal precautions seem adequate [48]. Instruments and contaminated areas should be disinfected with a sporicidal agent or 0.5% sodium hypochlorite solution [33]. Anthrax spores are highly resistant to drying and boiling for 10 minutes, and they resist most disinfectants. A temperature of 120°C for at least 15 minutes is normally used to inactivate the spores [50]. There are no specific recommendations on antibiotic prophylaxis or vaccination for health care workers exposed to patients with anthrax [48]. Decontamination of patients with soap and water is sufficient to reduce the possibility of secondary aerosolization of the spores.

*Anthrax as a weapon.* "Weaponized" anthrax refers to spores that have been milled, filtered, and coated to maximize their ability to disperse in the air, remain airborne, and deposit deep into the lungs [74]. A World Health Organization report estimated that the release of 50 kg of anthrax spores along a 2-km line upwind of a city of 500,000 people would result in 125,000 infections and 95,000 deaths. In 2001, the United States suffered a bioterrorist attack that resulted in the first ten confirmed cases of inhalational anthrax caused by the intentional release of *B anthracis*. Outbreaks occurred in the District of Columbia, Florida, New Jersey, and New York. As of November 7, 2001, a total of 22 cases of anthrax have been identified according to the CDC case definition (10 confirmed inhalational, 12 cutaneous). Five of the patients died.

*Plague*

*History.* At least three pandemics of plague have occurred in the sixth, fourteenth, and nineteenth centuries. The second pandemic in fourteenth-century Europe is often referred to as "the Black Death." At the peak of the last pandemic, plague was reported on every continent except Australia and Antarctica. It is believed that the three pandemics resulted in 200 million deaths [78,79]. In 1966, Viet Nam became the leading country for plague [80]. Destruction of the Vietnamese countryside and disruption of the ecosystem forced plague vectors into urban areas and led to the epidemic. US troops were not affected significantly.

*Epidemiology.* Plague remains an enzootic infection of rats, ground squirrels, prairie dogs, chipmunks, bobcats, and other rodents [79]. Human cases in the United States occur mainly in two regions: the Southwest (ie, Arizona, Colorado, Utah, New Mexico) and the Pacific region (ie, California, Oregon, Nevada). The first reported case in the United States was in San Francisco in 1900, and the last epidemic occurred in Los Angeles in 1924–1925. The 1924 epidemic is the last known human-to-human transmission in the United States [80]. There have been approximately 12 cases per year in the United States over the last two decades. The World Health Organization reports between 1000 and 3000 cases worldwide each year. There are three main clinical types of human plague: (1) bubonic, (2) septicemic, and (3) pneumonic [81].

*Microbiology.* *Y pestis* is an aerobic gram-negative, non–spore-forming, nonmotile bacillus of the family *Enterobacteriaceae* [79–83]. It demonstrates bipolar staining (closed safety pin appearance) with Giemsa, Wright's, and Wayson's stains. The characteristic bipolar staining is typically not evident on Gram stain. Colonies are pinpoint gray-white and are nonhemolytic on sheep blood agar [82]. It has the appearance of beaten copper on blood or McConkey's agar [80]. It is catalase positive and oxidase and urease negative. It does not ferment lactose. Its optimal growth temperature is room temperature (28°C) [82]. It may exhibit some degree of pleomorphism if grown on unfavorable media [81].

*Pathogenesis and clinical presentation.* Plague is primarily transmitted through the bite of the rodent flea, *Xenopsylla cheopis* (Oriental rat flea). The flea ingests a blood meal from an infected animal. The bacteria multiply in the flea's gut, and the infected flea regurgitates the organism into future victims [80]. Fleas generally prefer the rodent vector to humans and typically only leave dead rodents for humans in an attempt to continue their life cycle. *Y pestis* is a hardy bacteria and is able to withstand desiccation remarkably well compared with vegetative forms of other bacteria [80,81]. *Y pestis* can survive up to 3 days at room temperature, 3 weeks on dried blood, 5 weeks in flea species, and 11 months in rat burrows [79]. Once the vector bites the host, inoculation of up to 1000 organisms occurs [83]. The bacteria migrate by cutaneous lymphatics to the regional lymph nodes. Virulence is related to several antigens. Fraction I is an envelope antigen and is subjected to phagocytosis. If the bacterium is not killed by host defenses, it proliferates within the macrophages with the aid of Fraction I [80]. V and W antigens are also antiphagocytic but are related to virulence in an unknown manner. The lipopolysaccharide endotoxin moiety of the cell wall is similar to that found in other gram-negative bacilli [81]. Initially, the infection is contained within the regional lymph nodes, which causes lymphadenitis (the origin of the term "bubo" and thus, bubonic plague). The endotoxin is responsible for the septic state and resistance to host defenses [80]. The exotoxin, coagulase, seems to block the proventricular alimentary organ of the flea. This action prevents the flea from completely ingesting the blood meal, which results in delivery of the bacteria to the next host bitten [81]. Finally, there is mention of a plasminogen activator protein, which results in activation of the clotting cascade, possibly results in disseminated intravascular coagulation [81], and causes acral cyanosis and necrosis [80,83].

Bubonic plague typically follows a course as mentioned earlier. Illness typically begins after an incubation period of 2 to 8 days. Patients experience a sudden onset of fever, chills, weakness, headache, prostration, profound malaise, and enlarged, tender lymph nodes (buboes) [81], which typically occur in the groin, axilla, or cervical region [83]. The lymph nodes are so tender that patients resist movement. The skin overlying the nodes may be discolored or erythematous. Rarely the buboes may become fluctuant and suppurate [83]. Vital signs show fevers as high as 41°C, with an appropriate tachycardia for the increase in temperature. Blood pressure may be normal or low. Hypotension presumably results secondary to the "sepsis syndrome" [83]. Occasionally, patients present with lymphadenopathy without systemic signs and symptoms. These patients have a more favorable outcome.

Septicemic plague can occur as a primary form or as a secondary form via hematogenous spread of bubonic or pneumonic plague [80,84]. The primary form is a diagnostic challenge because it lacks the hallmark feature, the bubo. The clinical symptoms of fever, chills, nausea, vomiting, and hypotension are consistent with those seen in gram-negative sepsis. Acral cyanosis (believed to be the origin of "the Black Death"), disseminated intravascular coagulation, and purpura also may be seen. Severe abdominal pain is reported more often with the primary form [80].

Pneumonic plague rarely occurs as a primary form via inhalation of the organism from an aerosolized droplet nuclei from an infected patient or from aerosolized rodent fecal matter. The secondary form, which is more common, occurs via hematogenous spread of bubonic plague to the lungs [82]. Pneumonic plague is highly contagious. The incubation period is generally short—1 to 6 days. There is a rapid onset of tachycardia, fever, chest pain, dyspnea, cyanosis, and cough, which may produce bloody, purulent, or watery sputum [80]. Pleural effusions are common. The clinical course of pneumonic plague can progress rapidly to shock and multiorgan system failure and death [82].

Plague meningitis is an uncommon complication of other forms of plague and rarely can be the primary presentation [80]. Typically, it occurs more than 1 week after inadequately treated bubonic plague and is more often seen in association with axillary buboes. The bacteria possibly disseminate by direct lymphatic spread to the meninges. Clinical presentation is similar to any other form of bacterial meningitis and includes headache, fever, and meningismus. It is recommended that any CNS complaint be evaluated promptly [80].

*Diagnosis.* Three blood cultures drawn over a 45-minute period before beginning antimicrobial treatment generally provide a diagnosis. Growth invariably occurs within 48 hours. Bacterial isolation also can be accomplished with bubo aspirates and sputum cultures. Giemsa, Wright's, or Wayson's staining demonstrates the classic bipolar appearance. Serology is useful. A fourfold or more titer change or a single titer more than 1:28 to Fraction I antigen by passive hemagglutination testing also provides a diagnosis [81]. A single titer of 1:16 in unvaccinated patients is presumptive evidence of infection. ELISA to detect antibodies to Fraction I is more sensitive and specific than passive hemagglutination. ELISA is especially useful in diagnosing infection after antibiotics have been given [82]. The 5' nuclease PCR assay uses a fluorescently labeled oligonucleotide probe to detect and quantitate DNA templates rapidly in clinical samples. The PCR assay is 100% species specific and is sensitive to the picogram level [85]. A rapid immunogold dipstick chromatographic analysis to detect Fraction I has a specificity of 100% [86]. Mediastinal lymphadenopathy is rare on chest radiography and distinguishes plague from anthrax. Chest radiographs often show bilateral infiltrates, lobar consolidations, and pleural effusions. The differential diagnosis for plague includes tularemia, cat scratch disease, tuberculosis, chancroid, lymphogranuloma venereum, suppurative adenitis, and scrub typhus [80].

*Treatment.* Untreated bubonic plague has an estimated mortality rate of 50% [87]. Mortality rate in untreated pneumonic plague approaches 100% if appropriate antibiotics are not started within 24 hours [81]. The following recommendations come from the Working Group [88]. In contained casualty situations the treatment of choice for adults is streptomycin, 1 g intramuscularly (IM) twice a day, or gentamicin, 5 mg/kg IM/intravenously (IV) every day. Alternatives include doxycycline, 100 mg IV twice a day, ciprofloxacin, 400 mg IV twice a day, or chloramphenicol, 25 mg/kg IV four times a day. In children, the treatment of choice is streptomycin, 15 mg/kg IM twice a day (maximum dose, 2 g/d), or gentamicin, 2.5 mg/kg IM/IV three times a day. Alternatives include doxycycline, 2.2 mg/kg IV twice a day (maximum dose, 100 mg twice a day), ciprofloxacin, 15 mg/kg IV twice a day (maximum dose, 400 mg twice a day), or chloramphenicol, 25 mg/kg IV four times a day. In mass casualty situations, in which time would be compressed and supplies low, or for post-exposure prophylaxis, the Working Group recommends the following regimens. The recommended treatment for adults includes doxycycline, 100 mg orally twice a day, ciprofloxacin, 500 mg orally twice a day, or chloramphenicol, 25 mg/kg orally four times a day. The recommended treatment for children is doxycycline, 2.2 mg/kg orally twice a day (maximum dose, 100 mg twice a day) or ciprofloxacin, 20 mg/kg orally twice a day (maximum dose, 500 mg twice a day). If a child is older than 2 years, the recommended dosage is chloramphenicol, 25 mg/kg orally four times a day. The recommended duration of treatment in a mass casualty situation is 10 days. The recommended duration of postexposure prophylaxis is 7 days.

*Infection control and prevention.* All patients who are suspected of having plague should be placed in negative-pressure respiratory isolation. Recommended antimicrobial therapy should be started immediately after the drawing of blood cultures. The duration of isolation after treatment begins is 2 days for non–pneumonic plague and 4 days for pneumonic plague [82,83]. It is conceivable that during a mass casualty situation after a bioterrorist event, patients with pneumonic plague would be quarantined together while on treatment and be asked to wear surgical masks. Universal precautions at a minimum are required for all patient contact [82], and a National Institute for Occupation Safety and Health (NIOSH)-approved N-95 mask would offer greater protection [81]. Aerosol-generating procedures, such as bone sawing associated with surgery or post-mortem examinations, are not recommended [88]. No licensed vaccine for pneumonic plague currently is available in the United States [88].

*Plague as a weapon.* The World Health Organization estimates that dissemination of 50 kg of aerosolized *Y pestis* over a population center of 5 million people would cause 150,000 infections and 36,000 deaths. [82,88]. The bacterium would remain viable as an aerosol for 1 hour for a distance up to 10 km. City inhabitants might panic and attempt to flee the area, which would spread the disease farther [88]. An intentional release of aerosolized plague may result in (1) an unusual clustering of pneumonia and severe gram-negative septicemia in people who attended a large gathering or public event, (2) notable absence of buboes in patients diagnosed with plague pneumonia, (3) occurrence of disease in areas in which plague is not known to be endemic, (4) occurrence in people without occupational or environmental risks for plague, and (5) no reports of unusual animal deaths, particularly rodents, preceding the event [82]. The Working Group recommended that once pneumonic plague cases were known or strongly suspected of occurring, anyone with a fever or cough in the presumed area of exposure should be treated immediately with antibiotics for presumptive pneumonic plague. Delaying treatment until confirmatory testing is performed is not recommended and would decrease survival greatly [88]. Clinical deterioration of patients despite early initiation of treatment could signal antibiotic resistance.

*Botulinum toxin*

*History.* Botulism gets its name from an outbreak of disease in Southern Germany in the late 1700s. The outbreak involved 13 people who had consumed portions of the same large sausage (*botulus* is the Latin word for sausage) [89,90]. A detailed description of the clinical findings of the disease was provided by Justinus Kerner in 1817 [90,91]. In 1897, Emile van Ermengem investigated an epidemic in Eleezelles, Belgium. He isolated anaerobic bacteria from contaminated food and then produced the disease in laboratory animals by injecting them with the toxin produced by the bacteria [90,91]. As the Working Group pointed out, "it is regrettable that botulinum toxin still needs to be considered as a bioweapon at the historic moment when it has become the first biological toxin to become licensed for treatment of human disease" [92].

*Epidemiology.* Approximately 110 US cases of botulism are reported to the CDC each year [93]. There are five recognized forms of botulism: (1) classic (food borne), (2) infant, (3) wound, (4) hidden, and (5) inadvertent [94]. Food-borne botulism is caused by the ingestion of *Clostridium botulinum*–tainted food, classically, improperly home-canned fruits and vegetables. Infant botulism occurs when an infant ingests spores (less likely vegetative cells), which in turn colonize the intestinal tract and produce toxin [93,95]. Hidden botulism is a diagnosis of exclusion upon completion of an investigation if no source of the toxin can be found. Inadvertent botu-

**Box 3. Clinical features of infant botulism**

Weakness/hypotonia
Poor oral feeding/weak sucking
Constipation
Reduced gagging or sucking reflex
Weak cry
Ventilatory (respiratory) difficulty
Swallowing difficulties
Poor head control
Facial weakness
Lethargy/somnolence
Irritability
Hyporeflexia
Ocular abnormalities (mydriasis, ptosis)
Dry mouth
Cardiovascular abnormalities (hypotension, tachycardia)
Neurogenic bladder
Seizures (rare)

*Data from* Caya JG. Clostridium botulinum and the ophthalmologist: a review of botulism, including biological warfare ramifications of botulinum toxin. Surv Ophthalmol 2001;46(1):25–34.

lism refers to botulism that occurs as a result of IM injections of botulinum toxin [94] or an occupational exposure in laboratory workers via inhalation, which is the basis for bioterrorist plots [96]. Since 1980, infant botulism has been the most common form of botulism reported in the United States, with most of the cases reported in California. The number of wound botulism cases is rising secondary to illicit drug use, particularly use of "black tar heroin" [93].

*Microbiology.* Botulinum toxin is produced by anaerobic, spore-forming, gram-positive bacteria, *C botulinum*. The toxin is the most poisonous substance known. Low acidity (pH >5), low oxygen, and high water content favor spore formation. The toxin is heat labile, with inactivation occurring at temperatures >85°C; however, the spores are relatively heat resistant and require temperatures >120°C to be killed [94]. There are eight immunologically distinct toxins: A, B, C1, C2, D, E, F, and G. Botulinum toxin is a dichain polypeptide that consists of a "heavy" chain connected to a "light" chain by a single disulfide bond. The toxin's light chain is a zinc-containing endopeptidase that blocks acetylcholine-containing vesicles from fusing with the terminal membrane of

the motor neuron, which results in flaccid muscle paralysis. Botulinum toxin must be absorbed into the circulation from either a mucosal surface or a wound because it does not penetrate intact skin [92]. Most cases of human botulism are caused by types A, B, and E [93]. Recovery time from type A is longer than that of type E [94].

*Pathogenesis and clinical presentation.* The lethal dose of type A toxin for a 70-kg human is estimated to be 0.09 to 0.15 μg IV/IM, 0.7 to 0.9 μg inhalationally, or 70 μg orally [92]. All forms of human botulism produce identical neurologic signs. The rapidity of onset and severity of paralysis are dose dependent [92]. Food-borne botulism may present with nausea, vomiting, abdominal cramps, or diarrhea. The initial symptomatology is noted within 12 to 72 hours. Cognitive and sensory functions are almost always completely spared [95]. Botulism is an acute, afebrile, symmetric, descending flaccid paralysis that always begins in the bulbar musculature [92]. Botulism invariably displays multiple cranial nerve palsies; it is not possible to have botulism without them (Box 3; Table 4) [96].

Table 4
Signs and symptoms of food-borne and wound botulism

| Organ or system | Sign or symptom |
| --- | --- |
| Eye | Eyelid ptosis |
| | Ophthalmoplegia |
| | Sluggish or fixed, dilated pupils |
| | Nystagmus |
| | Blurred vision |
| | Diplopia |
| | Photophobia |
| Gastrointestinal | Dry mouth |
| | Dysphagia |
| | Sore throat |
| | Dysphonia |
| | Abdominal pain/cramps |
| | Diarrhea |
| | Nausea/vomiting |
| | Constipation |
| | Decreased gag reflex |
| Other | Generalized weakness |
| | Urinary retention |
| | Dizziness/vertigo |
| | Ataxia |
| | Ventilatory problems |
| | Decreased or absent deep tendon reflexes |

*Data from* Caya JG. Clostridium botulinum and the ophthalmologist: a review of botulism, including biological warfare ramifications of botulinum toxin. Surv Ophthalmol 2001;46(1):25–34.

*Diagnosis.* The initial diagnosis is based on history and physical examination findings. The differential diagnosis for botulism in adults and non-infant children includes Guillain-Barré syndrome, Miller-Fisher variant of Guillain-Barré syndrome, myasthenia gravis, Eaton-Lambert syndrome, tick paralysis, medication effects, organophosphate poisoning, and nerve gas exposure. The differential diagnosis for infant botulism includes failure to thrive, sepsis, dehydration, and poliomyelitis. Guillain-Barré syndrome usually presents with an ascending paralysis, although the Miller-Fisher variant may present a more difficult diagnostic challenge. Some patients may show a beneficial response to anticholinesterase drugs, such as edrophonium, which is used to test for myasthenia gravis [94]. If botulism is suspected, samples of blood and a list of patient medications should be sent to the CDC or state public health department [97]. The laboratory performs a mouse bioassay to determine toxin type [93]. If a food-borne or infant case is suspected, suspect food items and the patient's blood and possibly stool also should be sent to the laboratory. Demonstration of toxin in serum, stool, and suspect foodstuff provides a diagnosis. A positive stool culture for *C botulinum* is also diagnostic. Wound botulism is diagnosed by demonstrating toxin in the wound and obtaining a positive culture for *C botulinum* [98]. Electromyographic studies can provide presumptive evidence of botulism [94].

*Treatment.* The mortality of botulism has decreased with modern critical care therapy. The paralysis of botulism may persist for weeks to months, with concurrent requirements for assisted ventilation, nutritional support, fluid management and treatment of complications. Although there is irreversible binding of toxin to presynaptic endplates with irreparable damage, axons do regenerate by sprouting new endplates if one can assist the patient through the acute phase [96]. Therapy consists of aggressive supportive care and passive immunizations with equine antitoxin. Antitoxin use requires early suspicion of botulism. Antitoxin neutralizes toxin that is circulating in the blood. Antitoxin does not reverse established paralysis. One should not delay antitoxin administration for microbiologic testing [92,94]. In the United States there are two antitoxins—a trivalent antitoxin for neutralizing types A, B, and E and a heptavalent antitoxin available from USAMRIID under an investigational new drug protocol [92]. The dose of the trivalent antitoxin is 10 mL, which contains 7500 U of type A, 5500 U of type B, and 8500 U of type E. Antibiotics and surgical débridement may be necessary in secondary infections or in wound botulism. It

is recommended that if antibiotics are given, clindamycin, polymyxin B, and aminoglycosides not be used secondary to intrinsic neuromuscular blocking properties [94,96]. The use of guanidine has been shown to improve ocular and limb muscle strength in some patients [94].

*Infection control and prevention.* Standard precautions are all that is required. In the event of a bioterrorist attack, skin and clothing should be washed with soap and water. Contaminated objects and surfaces should be cleaned with a solution of 0.1% sodium hypochlorite for 10 to 15 minutes [93].

*Botulism as a weapon.* During World War II, the US Office of Strategic Services developed a plan for Chinese prostitutes to assassinate high-ranking Japanese officers. The US Office of Strategic Services prepared small gelatin capsules that contained botulinum toxin. This incident raises two points: (1) botulism need not occur in epidemics when used as a bioweapon and (2) botulism in animals may be a sign of biologic warfare [99]. If used as a weapon of mass destruction (WMD), botulinum toxin most likely would be used in an aerosolized form. After the 1991 Persian Gulf War, Iraq admitted to United Nations inspectors that they had produced 19,000 L of toxin and loaded 10,000 L into weapons. These 19,000 L of toxin are not fully accounted for [92]. With most bioterrorist events, the aerosol dissemination may not be difficult to recognize secondary to a large number of cases sharing a common temporal and geographic exposure and lack a common dietary exposure. Identification of the exposure site initially may be difficult because of the mobility of people during the incubation phase [92]. There never have been any instances of water-borne botulism. It is unlikely that botulinum toxin would be used in a scenario involving contamination of a municipal water supply for two reasons. First, standard potable water treatment would inactivate the toxin. Second, a large inoculum of toxin would be necessary secondary to the slow turnover time of large capacity reservoirs. Botulinum toxin may be stable in untreated water for several days, however, and should be investigated when no other source of an outbreak can be identified [96].

*Tularemia*
*History.* Tularemia was first described in 1911 as a plague-like disease in rodents in Tulare County, California [100].

*Epidemiology.* In the United States, tularemia has occurred in every state except Hawaii [101,102]. *Francisella tularensis* is found in various terrestrial and aquatic mammals, including ground squirrels, rabbits, hares, voles, muskrats, and water rats. Human outbreaks of the disease parallel wild animal outbreaks. Arthropod vectors also have been implicated in the transmission of disease, including ticks and biting flies [103]. There is an average of 124 cases per year. Tularemia was removed from the list of reportable diseases in 1994 but was reinstated in 2000 because of bioterrorism concerns [104].

*Microbiology.* Tularemia is also known as rabbit fever or deer fly fever [105]. *F tularensis* is an aerobic, nonmotile, gram-negative coccobacillus. It is a hardy non–spore-forming organism with a thin lipopolysaccharide-containing envelope. It can survive for weeks at low temperatures and in water, moist soil, hay, and decaying animal carcasses [101]. There are two main subspecies: holarctica, which replaced palearctica and is less virulent, and tularensis, which is more virulent. There are three biovars of subspecies holarctica: erythromycin sensitive, erythromycin resistant, and japonica [103].

*Pathogenesis and clinical presentation.* Tularemia can be transmitted to humans by insect vectors, handling of infected animal tissue, ingestion of infected animal tissue, and contaminated water or inhalation of infectious aerosol [100]. *F tularensis* is a facultative intracellular bacterium that multiplies within macrophages. The major organs involved are the lymph nodes, lungs, liver, spleen, and kidneys. The initial tissue reaction is a focal, intensely suppurative necrosis that ultimately becomes granulomatous. Inhalational exposure results in hemorrhagic inflammation of the airways that may progress to bronchopneumonia [101]. As few as 10 to 15 organisms can cause disease [105]. Head and neck signs and symptoms are found in 11% to 45% of infected patients. There are seven clinical syndromes of tularemia: (1) ulceroglandular, 21% to 78% of cases; (2) glandular, 3% to 20% of cases; (3) oculoglandular, <5% of cases; (4) oropharyngeal <12% of cases; (5) pneumonic, 7% to 20% of cases; (6) typhoidal, 5% to 30% of cases; and (7) septic [106]. After a 1- to 21-day incubation period (average 3–5 days), there is an abrupt onset of fever, chills, myalgia, arthralgia, malaise, rhinorrhea, sore throat, and fatigue [101,107]. There may be a dry or slightly productive cough and substernal pain with or without signs of pneumonia, such as purulent sputum, dyspnea, tachypnea, pleuritic pain, and hemoptysis. A pulse–temperature dissociation frequently is seen. Nausea, vomiting, and diarrhea may occur. Hematogenous spread can complicate any form of tularemia and possibly result in meningitis, pericarditis, hepatitis, endocarditis, ataxia, osteomyelitis, sepsis, and acute renal failure [107].

In the ulceroglandular form, a tender or pruritic inflammatory papule develops at the site of inoculation, usually on the hands and distal extremities. The papule enlarges rapidly and is followed by a sharply demarcated ulcer with a thin, yellow exudate. A necrotic base and black eschar may form along with the onset of regional lymphadenopathy. The ulcer may persist for months and ultimately heals with scarring. The involved lymph nodes may become fluctuant and drain spontaneously. Secondary skin eruptions (tularemids) are common and occur in 3% to 25% of cases [108]. Tularemic exanthems appear most often during the second week of the disease. Erythema nodosum, erythema multiforme, and Sweet's syndrome also have been reported [107].

The glandular form is characterized by fever and tender lymphadenopathy in the absence of skin manifestations [106,107].

The oculoglandular form is characterized by painful, purulent, unilateral conjunctivitis with cervical and preauricular lymphadenopathy [107]. The preauricular lymphadenopathy serves to differentiate tularemia from cat scratch disease, tuberculosis, sporotrichosis, and syphilis [107,109]. The conjunctiva is the site of inoculation secondary to contact with contaminated fingers or infected matter. Patients may complain of photophobia, excessive lacrimation, lid edema, and conjunctivitis. Complications include corneal ulceration and dacryocystitis [106].

The oropharyngeal form results from ingestion of contaminated food or fluids. It is more common in children and may affect multiple family members [106]. Patients present with cervical lymphadenopathy, exudative or membranous pharyngitis, and tonsillitis. Patients complain of abdominal pain, nausea, vomiting, diarrhea, intestinal ulcerations, gastrointestinal bleeding, and mesenteric lymphadenopathy [107].

The typhoidal form is acquired from any form, but prominent lymphadenopathy or other localizing signs or symptoms are absent [106].

In the pneumonic form, primary pneumonic tularemia results from inhalation. Secondary pneumonic tularemia results from hematogenous spread from other forms. This form occurs most often in laboratory workers, farmers, and sheep shearers [106].

*Diagnosis.* For differential diagnoses, refer to Table 5. Tularemia would be expected to have a slower progression of illness and a lower case-fatality rate than inhalational plague or anthrax [101]. Histopathologic testing of the ulcer demonstrates a granulomatous reaction that may be tuberculoid in appearance. The necrosis is more liquefactive than caseating. The widespread necrosis is characterized by leukocytes, lymphocytes, and multinucleated giant cells surrounded by epithelioid cells and fibrosis [100]. Imaging features are nonspecific, and Gram stain is of little value. The definitive diagnosis is a positive culture from sputum, blood, ulcer and eye exudates, pharyngeal washings, and fasting gastric aspirates [101,105]. The organism has been demonstrated in pleural biopsy using the glucose oxidase immunoenzyme staining technique [105]. Agglutination titers with a fourfold increase are diagnostic; a single titer more than 1:160 is presumptive of tularemia. Antibody titers reach a maximum level at 4 to 8 weeks and may remain detectable for years after infection.

*Treatment.* Mortality rates from biovar tularensis are in the range of 5% to 15%. Currently, the overall fatality rate in the United States is <2%. Biovar holarctica infections are rarely fatal [101,103]. The Working Group recommends the following antibiotic therapy for contained casualty situations. The recommended regimen for adults is streptomycin, 1g IM twice a day, or gentamicin, 5 mg/kg IM/IV every day. Alternatively, the regimen is doxycycline, 100 mg IV twice a day, chloramphenicol, 15 mg/kg IV four times a day, or ciprofloxacin, 400 mg IV twice a day. For pregnant women, the preferred regimen is gentamicin, 5 mg/kg IM/IV every day or streptomycin, 1g IM twice a day, or alternatively, doxycycline, 100 mg IV twice a day, or ciprofloxacin, 400 mg IV twice a day. For children, the preferred regimen is streptomycin, 15 mg/kg IM twice a day (maximum dose, 2 g/d), or gentamicin, 2.5 mg/kg IM/IV three times a day, or alternatively doxycycline, 2.2 mg/kg IV twice a day (maximum dose, 100 mg twice a day), or chloramphenicol, 15 mg/kg IV four times a day, or ciprofloxacin, 15 mg/kg IV twice a day (maximum dose, 400 mg twice a day). In a mass casualty situation, the Working Group recommends the following regimens. The preferred adult regimen is doxycycline, 100 mg orally twice a day, or ciprofloxacin, 500 mg orally twice a day. The preferred children's regimen is doxycycline, 2.2 mg/kg orally twice a day (maximum dose, 100 mg twice a day), or ciprofloxacin, 15 mg/ kg orally twice a day (maximum dose, 500 mg twice a day). The recommended regimen for pregnant women is ciprofloxacin, 500 mg orally twice a day, or doxycycline, 100 mg orally twice a day. Antibiotic susceptibility testing should be performed as soon as possible. Treatment with aminoglycosides or ciprofloxacin should continue for 10 days. Treatment with chloramphenicol or doxycycline should continue for 14 days because of a higher relapse or treatment failure rate [101].

*Infection control and prevention.* Transmission between humans occurs occasionally [100]. The Working Group does not recommend isolation for infected patients. Standard precautions are recommended. Procedures likely to generate aerosols are not recommended. Decontamination can be achieved with a 10% hypochlorite solution after 10 minutes; 70% alcohol solution can be used to clean the area further. In the event of a bioterrorist attack, it is

Table 5
Differential diagnoses of different forms of tularemia

| Type | Differential diagnosis |
| --- | --- |
| Ulceroglandular | Anthrax, sporotrichosis, nontuberculous mycobacterial infection, deep fungal infection, brown recluse spider bite, cutaneous leishmaniasis, glanders, plague |
| Oculoglandular | Pyogenic bacterial infection, syphilis, herpes zoster, adenoviral infection, cat scratch disease, sporotrichosis, anthrax, scrub typhus, rat bite fever, streptococcal or staphylococcal lymphadenitis |
| Oropharyngeal | Streptococcal pharyngitis, mononucleosis, diphtheria, viral pharyngitis, cat scratch disease, anthrax, plague, lyme disease, tuberculosis, lymphoma, leukemia |
| Pneumonic | Atypical pneumonia, chlamydia pneumonia, Q fever, sarcoidosis, mycoplasma, psittacosis, histoplasmosis, coccidiomycosis |
| Typhoidal | Typhoid fever, brucellosis, tuberculosis, malaria, Legionnaire's disease, psittacosis, Q fever, sarcoidosis, reticuloendothelial or hematologic malignancies |

*Data from* Rinaldo A, Bradley PJ, Ferlito A. Tularemia in otolaryngology: a forgotten but not gone disease and a possible sign of bio-terrorism. J Laryngol Otol 2004;118(4):257–9; Greenfield RA, Drevets DA, Machado LJ, et al. Bacterial pathogens as biological weapons and agents of bioterrorism. Am J Med Sci 2002;323(6):299–315; Cronquist SD. Tularemia: the disease and the weapon. Dermatol Clin 2004;22(3):313–20.

recommended that people avoid sick or dead animals. A live attenuated vaccine is recommended for laboratory workers only, although this is under review by the US Food and Drug Administration [101].

*Tularemia as a weapon.* It has been suggested that the Soviet Army used tularemia as a biologic weapon during the Battle of Stalingrad [110]. In 1969, the World Health Organization estimated that a 50-kg aerosol dispersal of virulent *F tularensis* over a city with a population of 5 million would result in 250,000 incapacitating injuries and 19,000 deaths. Referring to this model, the CDC estimated the economic impact of such an attack to be $5.4 billion/100,000 people exposed.

## Viral hemorrhagic fevers

*History.* Viral hemorrhagic fever (VHF) denotes a clinical syndrome characterized by fever and a bleeding diathesis that results from an infection by a virus that belongs to any of the following virus families: *Filoviridae, Arenaviridae, Flaviviridae*, or *Bunyaviridae* [111]. It is possible that the Great Plagues of Athens (430–427/425 BC) described by Thucydides were outbreaks of VHF [111]. Marburg, the first filovirus described, was identified in 1967 after a cluster of hemorrhagic fever cases occurred in laboratory workers in Marburg, Germany. Ebola virus was named after a river in former Zaire (Democratic Republic of Congo). In 1989, Ebola was found in the United States in quarantined monkeys from the Philippines. The most recent strain was identified in 1994 in Cote d'Ivoire after an autopsy on an infected chimpanzee [112].

*Virology.* Ebola and Marburg viruses belong to the family *Filoviridae*. Junin virus (Argentine hemorrhagic fever), Machupa virus (Bolivian hemorrhagic fever), Sabia virus (Brazillian hemorrhagic fever), and arenavirus (Lassa fever) belong to the family *Arenaviridae*. Hanta virus, Nairovirus (Crimean Congo hemorrhagic fever), and phlebovirus (Rift Valley fever) belong to the family *Bunyaviridae*. Yellow fever and dengue fever belong to the family *Flaviviridae*. All of the VHFs are lipid-enveloped RNA viruses that require an animal or insect host reservoir [113]. Transmission of VHF occurs through contact with infected persons or nonhuman primate body fluids. Fomites may be sources of transmission because filoviruses retain their infectivity on environmental surfaces while at room temperature [114]. The particular reservoir of the filoviruses is yet to be identified [112].

*Pathogenesis and clinical presentation.* As a group, agents of VHF spread hematogenously to multiple organs and target the vascular endothelium, which causes microvascular damage and marked changes in vascular permeability. Primary viral replication occurs in cells of the mononuclear phagocyte system, particularly those in the liver, spleen, lymph nodes, lungs, and bone marrow, which allows for evasion from the immune system and amplification of the infection [111]. Severe manifestations of infection result from the interplay of vascular permeability, proinflammatory cytokine release, cytotoxic factors, autoantibodies, complement activation, and systemic coagulopathy [113]. The clinical situation progresses to shock and death secondary to increased vascular permeability, intravascular volume loss, and multiorgan failure. Filoviruses are the most destructive of the VHFs, with widespread necrosis of internal organs, hemorrhages, and ecchymosis. The necrosis is ischemic and cytopathic [111]. Incubation periods vary from 2 to 19 days and lead to initial, abrupt onset of fever, myalgia, pain, and prostration [113]. Patients may have conjunctival injection, hypotension, flushing, and petechial hemorrhages on examination. Hemorrhage may be in the form of hematemesis, melena, or hematuria and is associated with a poor prognosis, although not all patients with bleeding die. Survivors from the 1967 Marburg outbreak revealed no long-term sequelae, and most of them returned to work within 3 months of recovery [115].

*Diagnosis.* The differential diagnosis of VHFs includes malaria, meningococcemia, rickettsial diseases, leptospirosis, typhoid fever, dysentery, plague, and hemorrhagic smallpox. Tests for VHF must be performed in a biosafety level 4 laboratory (USAMRIID or CDC). Specimens should be double bagged and pretreated with Triton X-100 before analysis. Immediate diagnosis strategies include RT-PCR, antigen detection, and viral isolation. ELISA techniques are more useful once an epidemic has been identified [111].

*Treatment.* The overall mortality rate for Ebola virus is between 53% and 88%; for Marburg virus it is between 23% and 84% [112]. The typical disease course lasts 10 to 14 days, with fatalities occurring between 7 and 11 days [111]. The management of any VHF is aggressive critical care, including vigilant attention to fluid and electrolyte status, nutrition, and pressor support. Ribavarin has been shown to reduce mortality in Lassa fever and other Arenaviruses, but it plays no role in the treatment of Ebola virus. Novel treatments are being attempted but are of limited or unknown value. These treatments include use of polyclonal equine hyperimmune sera, neutralizing human monoclonal antibodies, murine monoclonal antibodies, use of whole-blood transfusions derived from Ebola survivors (Ebola specific), new pharmacotherapies, carbocyclic 3-deazaadenosine, and a new vaccine currently in a phase I trial.

*Infection control and prevention.* Ebola virus is stable at room temperature and can withstand desiccation. The virus can be inactivated in 30 minutes at 60°C, and infectivity can be diminished greatly by gamma irradiation, ultraviolet light in high doses, and lipid solvents in phenolic disinfectants [111]. Patients with suspected infections or known infections should be placed in private respiratory isolation rooms with negative-pressure and an anteroom. The number of staff and visitors should be restricted because all contacts must be monitored for 21 days after exposure. It is recommended that patients have single-use equipment. Contact and droplet precautions should be followed, and in addition to universal precautions an N-95 mask is recommended. All linen should be double bagged, washed without sorting in hot water with bleach, autoclaved, or incinerated. Cadavers should not be embalmed [111]. For survivors, Ebola virus has been detected in vaginal secretions and semen up to 3 months after infection. It is recommended that people use condoms for at least 3 months after recovery [112].

*Viral hemorrhagic fevers as a weapon.* The Soviet Union produced Marburg, Ebola, Lassa, Junin, and Machupa viruses in large quantities for use as biologic weapons [112]. These viruses pose a serious risk because of the following characteristics: (1) low infectious dose, (2) easy dissemination via an aerosol, (3) lack of effective vaccine, (4) availability for procurement, (5) ability to be produced in large quantities, (6) relative stability in the environment, and (7) previous use as a weapon [12]. Although they are the archetypical diseases of VHFs, yellow fever and dengue fever are not significant biologic weapons threats [33].

## Category B

### Q fever
*History.* In 1937, Edward Derrick first described a febrile illness that affected abattoir workers in Australia, which he termed Q (for Query) fever because of the uncertain nature of the disease [116]. In 1944–1945, American and British troops in Florence, Italy

suffered a severe outbreak; over a 3-week period more than 300 soldiers (one third of the 900 troops stationed there) developed Q fever, as did 20 people in the laboratory in Naples, Italy that handled the specimens. No deaths occurred, but 1000 cases were diagnosed [117]. Q fever was identified in the United States in 1939 during investigations into the causal agent for the so-called 9-mile fever in Montana [116].

*Epidemiology.* Q fever is a worldwide zoonotic disease caused by *Coxiella burnetii*. The most common animal reservoirs are cattle, sheep, and goats; infected animals are usually asymptomatic. The placenta of infected animals is usually heavily contaminated (up to $10^9$ organisms/g in sheep) and at parturition results in environmental contamination [106]. Humans, however, seem to be the only hosts who manifest disease as a result of infection [118]. Human infection typically follows inhalation of aerosolized bacteria. *C burnetii* is virulent, with disease being caused by as few as 1 to 10 organisms [106, 116,118]. Sheep represent one of the largest sources of human exposure. In the rural setting, the exposure may be manure contaminated with products of conception/parturition, dust produced in the shearing of wool contaminated with tick feces, secondary aerosolization via herding animals, or wind [117]. Air samples are positive for up to 2 weeks after parturition [106]. In the urban setting, infection results from exposure to commercial slaughter houses, infected cats, dogs, or rats, or rarely, ingestion of contaminated dairy products [116]. The true incidence of Q fever is unknown because of asymptomatic cases and the underreporting of febrile, flu-like illnesses.

*Microbiology.* Historically, *C burnetii* was named *Rickettsia diaporica* and *Rickettsia burnetii*. Gene sequence analysis classifies the organism in the order *Legionella*. The organism is a pleomorphic, gram-variable coccobacillus [116]. The organism is an obligate intracellular rickettsia-like bacterium that lives and proliferates in acidic phagolysosomes [117]. In adverse environments it produces a spore-like form termed small-cell variant [119]. These small-cell variants have a thickened cell wall and are metabolically inactive. They become activated only after phagolysosomal fusion causes acid activation of the cell [117]. The small-cell variants are resistant to heat, cold, desiccation, fixation in formaldehyde, and fixation in paraffinized tissue blocks [106]. The key feature that determines the organism's virulence is the lipopolysaccharide on its outer surface [117].

*C burnetii* is generally of low virulence but high infectivity [105].

*Pathogenesis and clinical presentation.*     Although humoral and cell-mediated immunity plays a role in controlling infection, cell-mediated immunity seems ultimately to eliminate the organism [116]. Once infected, a transient bacteremia occurs followed by dissemination to the liver and other organs, including the genitourinary tract [117]. T-cell and macrophage function are impaired. The suppression of antimicrobial function allows for the persistence and intracellular multiplication of the organisms. An intact T-cell–mediated immune response is required for containment of the infection. There are reports that despite most initial infections being controlled, reactivation or exacerbation of disease can occur in patients who later become immunosuppressed. This reactivation/exacerbation suggests that the organism lingers as a latent infection. An adequate T-cell response to infection results in granuloma formation. If the infection is not contained by the immune system, a chronic infection can result [117]. The incubation period ranges from 14 to 26 days (average, 15 days). The initial presentation may be a flu-like illness, atypical pneumonia, or hepatitis [117]. The flu-like syndrome is self-limiting and lasts 1 to 2 weeks. The symptoms include a sudden-onset high fever, nausea, fatigue, headache, myalgia, chills, and photophobia [106,116]. A person may experience a 6- to 12-kg weight loss [120]. Pneumonia is common. It occurs in 50% of cases and is often an incidental radiographic finding. Hepatitis is also a common occurrence (33% of cases), and it may be symptomatic or clinically silent [106,116]. Liver cell necrosis with granulomata occurs in severe cases [116]. Chronic manifestations of Q fever can include malaise similar to chronic fatigue syndrome, endocarditis, granulomatous hepatitis, aseptic meningitis, and encephalitis [106].

*Diagnosis.*     The diagnosis of Q fever depends on serologic testing. Indirect fluorescent antibody ELISA and PCR techniques are useful [121]. All serologic techniques have cross-reactions to *Legionella* and *Bartonella* species.

*Treatment.*     The overall mortality rate of Q fever is 1% to 2%. Patients with acute Q fever may develop the chronic form in 1 to 20 years [106]. The recommended treatment is as follows [116,117]: for adults, tetracycline, 500 mg orally every 6 hours for 2 weeks, or doxycycline, 100 mg orally/IV twice a day for 2 to 3 weeks. For children, the recommended treatment is trimethoprim/sulfamethoxazole, 2.2 to 4 mg/kg of trimethoprim, orally/IV twice a day for 2 to 3 weeks, or chloramphenicol, 25 mg/kg orally twice a day. Q fever endocarditis is difficult to treat and requires at least 2 years of treatment with a tetracycline combined with rifampin or fluoroquinolone or hydroxychloroquine. Hydroxychloroquine is recommended to increase the alkalinization of the phagolysosome (from pH 4.8 to 5.7) and the intracellular action of doxycycline. Suggested regimens include (1) doxycycline, 100 mg orally twice a day, and hydroxychloroquine, 200 mg orally every 8 hours for 18 to 24 months, or (2) doxycycline, 100 mg orally twice a day, and ofloxacin, 200 mg orally every 8 hours for 3 to 4 years. Valvular replacement is frequently required. Postexposure prophylaxis is the same as for disease treatment, but the duration of therapy is only 5 to 7 days [117].

*Infection control and prevention.*     Human-to-human transmission does not seem to occur. Specimens should be processed under biosafety level 3 conditions. Obstetric procedures should be performed under aerosol/droplet precaution conditions [121]. Decontamination with soap and water is sufficient. Effective disinfectant solutions include a 30-minute exposure to 70% ethanol, 5% chloroform, or 2.25% N-alkyldimethyl benzyl and 2.25% ethylbenzal ammonium chloride (5% Enviro-Chem, Chem Sales, Ellicott City, Maryland) [117]. A formalin-killed vaccine (Q-vax) is licensed in Australia with documented immunity lasting at least 5 years [118]. All Q fever vaccines in the United States are investigational [105].

*Q fever as a weapon.*     It is estimated that a 50-kg *C burnetii* aerosol release along a 2-km line upwind from a city with a population of 500,000 would reach areas more than 20 km away and would cause 150 deaths, 125,000 incapacitated patients, and 9000 cases of Q fever endocarditis [122].

### Brucellosis
*History.*     A British Army surgeon described a chronic relapsing illness on the island of Minorca in the Mediterranean. In 1887, Sir David Bruce isolated the causative organism. In 1897, M.L. Hughes published detailed clinical and pathologic findings and called the disease undulant fever. Also in 1897, B. Bang, a Dane, identified an organism that caused contagious abortion and called it bacillus of abortion. The first US case was reported in 1898. In 1917, another investigator, Evans, recognized that Bang's organism was identical to that of Bruce's organism [123].

*Epidemiology.* Brucellosis is a worldwide zoonotic infection. Transmission occurs from animals to humans via ingestion of infected animal food products, direct or indirect contact with an infected animal, or inhalation of infectious aerosols [123]. Brucellosis in the United States occurs in 0.5/100,000 population, with most cases reported in California, Florida, Texas, and Virginia. During the past 10 years, approximately 100 cases were reported in the United States. Most US cases were secondary to ingestion of infected milk or dairy products [124].

*Microbiology.* Brucellae are small, slow-growing, aerobic, gram-negative, nonmotile, non–spore-forming unencapsulated coccobacilli [106,121,123]. The organisms are facultative intracellular macrophage parasites and localize in the lung, spleen, liver, CNS, bone marrow, and synovium [105]. Four of six species of *Brucellae* (in order of pathogenicity) are important pathogens in humans: (1) *B melitensis* (goats), (2) *B suis* (swine), (3) *B abortus* (cattle), and (4) *B canis* (dog) [123].

*Pathogenesis and clinical presentation.* Inhalation of 10 to 100 bacteria can produce human infection [106]. The incubation period is 1 to 8 weeks [123]. Smooth cell wall lipopolysaccharide is the principle virulence factor that enables resistance to intracellular killing by leukocytes [125]. Production of adenine and guanine monophosphate contributes to intracellular survival by inhibiting degranulation of polymorphonuclear leukocytes and suppressing the myeloperoxidase-hydrogen peroxide-halide system and a copper zinc superoxide dismutase. The principle recovery mechanism is T-cell–mediated immunity [106]. Survival within macrophages is the probable basis for chronic infection. Intracellular survival is also believed to be heme dependent. *Brucellae* species use ferrochelatase to synthesize their own heme stores. Many systems can be involved with brucellosis, including dermal, neurologic, respiratory, gastrointestinal, genitourinary, hematologic, osteoarticular, renal, and cardiovascular [105,125]. The clinical signs of an infection are the same regardless of the route of exposure [105] and may manifest as acute, subacute, or chronic forms. The acute form occurs within 8 weeks of exposure and is associated with flu-like symptoms (ie, fever, chills, sweats, malaise, anorexia, headache, myalgias, and back pain). The subacute form or undulant form usually occurs within 12 months of exposure and is associated with undulant fevers, arthritis, and orchi-epididymitis. The chronic form occurs after 12 months from exposure and is associated with chronic fatigue, depression, weight loss, and arthritis. Other signs and symptoms include irritability, depression, mental status changes, nuchal rigidity, seizures, coma, uveitis, optic neuritis, papilledema, arthralgias, arthritis, spondylitis, sacroiliitis, vertebral osteomyelitis, anemia, neutropenia, thrombocytopenia, and granulomatous hepatitis [105,106,123]. Rarely, endocarditis, aortitis, and aortic aneurysms may occur. Pulmonary complaints are also uncommon and manifest as a nonproductive cough, pleuritic chest pain, and, rarely, pleural effusions [105,106,121,123,125].

*Diagnosis.* Brucellosis is notoriously difficult to diagnose [123]. The differential diagnosis includes Q fever, salmonella, tularemia, syphilis, tuberculosis, histoplasmosis, sarcoidosis, and lymphoma. Blood cultures and bone marrow aspirates are the standard tests used to isolate the bacteria [125]. Cultures should be held for 4 to 6 weeks [105,121]. Results of a serum agglutination test are positive with seroconversion or titer ≥1:160 [105]. ELISA and PCR techniques are available [105,125].

*Treatment.* Table 6 lists treatment regimens [105, 106,123,125,126].

*Infection control and prevention.* Isolation is not required because of a low to zero incidence of human-to-human transmission. Contact precautions should be used for patients with open wounds. There is no effective human vaccine [121], although animal vaccines have eliminated most disease among domesticated animals in the United States [105,125]. Brucella may survive up to 6 weeks in dust and 10 weeks in soil and water, which leads to the potential risk of re-aerosolization. Brucella are susceptible to disinfectants and heat, so routine decontamination with soap and water is recommended [123]. Autoclaving of linen and clothes is recommended. Specimens should be handled in a biosafety level 3 laboratory [123].

*Brucella as a weapon.* *Brucella* species became the first agent to be weaponized in the United States [123]. The economic impact estimates for a bioterrorist attack with brucella are $478 million/100,000 people exposed [121]. If a population center of 100,000 people was exposed to a brucella bioterrorist attack, 82,500 cases of disease and 413 deaths would be expected [123].

### Ricin

*History and toxicology.* Worldwide, 1 million tons of castor beans are processed annually. Ricin is a

Table 6
World Health Organization recommended treatment for brucellosis

| Category | Preferred | Duration | Alternative | Duration |
|---|---|---|---|---|
| Adult | Doxycycline, 100 mg orally twice a day and Rifampin, 600–900 mg orally every day | 6 wk | Doxycycline, 100 mg orally twice a day and Streptomycin, 1 g IV/IM every day or | 2–6 wk |
| | | | Gentamycin, 5 mg/kg IV/IM every day or | 1–3 wk |
| | | | Trimethoprim/sulfamethoxazole, 160 mg/800 mg orally twice a day or 8–10 mg/kg IV or | 6 wk |
| | | | Ciprofloxacin, 500 mg orally twice a day and Rifampin, 600 mg orally every day | 4 wk |
| Children <8 y | Rifampin, 10–20 mg/kg oral/IV (maximum dose, 600 mg) and Trimethoprim/sulfamethoxazole, 40 mg/200 mg/10 kg orally (maximum dose, 160 mg/800 mg) | 6 wk | Rifampin, 10–20 mg/kg oral/IV (maximum dose, 600 mg) and Gentamycin, 5 mg/kg IM every day or | 1 wk |
| | | | Trimethoprim/sulfamethoxazole, 40 mg/200 mg/10kg orally (maximum dose, 160 mg/800 mg) and Streptomycin, 20–40 mg/kg IM every day (maximum dose, 1 g/d) or | 6 wk |
| | | | Gentamycin, 5 mg/kg IM every day | 5 d |
| Children >8 y | Doxycycline, 100 mg orally twice a day and Streptomycin, 1 g IV every day or Gentamycin, 5 mg/kg IM every day | 6 wk 2 wk 1 wk | Doxycycline, 100 mg orally twice a day and Rifampin, 10–20 mg/kg oral/IV (maximum dose, 600 mg) or | 6 wk |
| | | | Trimethoprim/sulfamethoxazole, 40 mg/200 mg/10 kg orally (maximum dose, 160 mg/800 mg) and Streptomycin, 20–40 mg/kg IM every day (maximum dose, 1 g/d) or | 6 wk 5 d |
| | | | Gentamycin, 5 mg/kg IM every day | |
| Pregnant Women | Rifampin, 600–900 mg orally every day | 6 wk | Rifampin, 900 mg orally every day and Trimethoprim/sulfamethoxazole, 160 mg/800 mg orally twice a day | 4 wk |
| Postexposure prophylaxis | Doxycycline, 100 mg orally twice a day and Rifampin, 600 mg orally every day | 3 wk | | |

Combination therapy is recommended secondary to high relapse rates and suboptimal results with monotherapy.
*Data from* Refs. [105,106,123,125,126].

protein (toxin) produced from the waste products of castor bean processing [127]. The waste mash contains a high concentration of ricin (5%) by weight. The lethal dose is approximately 5 μg/kg [128]. Separation of the toxin from the mash is not difficult and requires only undergraduate chemistry techniques [14]. Ricin is a relatively stable protein composed of two chains—A and B—linked by a disulfide bond. The B chain binds to cell surface receptors and is endocytosed. The A chain inhibits protein synthesis via inactivation of the 28S ribosomal RNA subunit [127–129].

*Pathogenesis and clinical presentation.* "Clinical manifestations of ricin intoxication vary with route of exposure" [129]. The oral route is the least toxic secondary to limited absorption and enzymatic degradation [14,128]; however, necrosis of the gastrointestinal tract occurs with gastrointestinal, splenic, hepatic, and renal hemorrhage [128,129]. Ricin is most toxic via inhalational exposure. After inhalation, there is an incubation period of 4 to 8 hours. Necrosis of respiratory epithelium occurs, with death resulting from respiratory failure caused by a capillary leak-like syndrome within 36 to 72 hours [14,128]. Ricin is a potent immunogen; survivors are likely to have high circulating antibody levels for several weeks after exposure [14]. Typical symptoms associated with ingestion appear in 1 to 4 hours and include nausea, vomiting, bloody or nonbloody diarrhea, and abdominal cramping. The diarrhea leads to substantial fluid loss, dehydration, and, ultimately, hypovolemic shock. If the case is severe, liver and renal failure and death may occur. Inhalational exposure to ricin causes fever, chest tightness, cough, dyspnea, nausea, arthralgias, and diaphoresis [130].

*Diagnosis.* The differential diagnosis includes any biologic agent that can produce acute respiratory disease (eg, staphylococcal enterotoxin B, mycotoxins, anthrax, tularemia, plague) [14]. There are no existing tests for the detection of ricin in biologic fluid [130].

*Treatment.* Treatment for ricin intoxication is supportive with aggressive critical care measures [14, 127,128,130]. There is no specific antidote, and the toxin is not removed by dialysis. The efficacy of gastric lavage is controversial. A single dose of activated charcoal should be administered as soon as possible if ricin intoxication is suspected and the patient is not vomiting. Ipecac, whole bowel irrigation, and other cathartics should not be used routinely [130].

*Infection control and prevention.* Decontamination with soap and water is sufficient. There is no vaccine for ricin intoxication. There is little risk for human-to-human transmission [121]. Re-aerosolization is a potential risk.

*Ricin as a weapon.* An outbreak of a large number of patients with an acute lung injury syndrome should suggest the possibility of an airborne ricin bioterrorist attack. Ricin could be used as a weapon via an aerosol or food contaminant. It is less likely that it would be used to contaminate water supplies because of its relatively low potency [128].

*Staphylococcal enterotoxin B*

*History and toxicology.* Staphylococcal enterotoxins are a superfamily of proteins (11 different serotypes) secreted by *Staphylococcus aureus* [128]. The toxins are most commonly associated with foodborne gastroenteritis, but they also can cause toxic shock syndrome, scalded skin syndrome, and bullous impetigo [14,127,128]. Staphylococcal enterotoxin B has two binding sites, a high affinity site for major histocompatibility complex II proteins, and a low affinity site for a T-cell receptor. T-cell receptor binding results in a massive release of pro-inflammatory cytokines. As little as 250 to 400 ng of the toxin can induce symptoms [127,128].

*Clinical presentation.* Staphylococcal enterotoxin B intoxication is more of an incapacitating agent. Symptoms occur 3 to 12 hours after exposure and include fever, headache, conjunctivitis, chills, nausea, vomiting, and diarrhea [14,127–129]. With severe intoxication, profound dehydration, shock, respiratory failure, and cardiovascular collapse may occur.

*Diagnosis.* The differential diagnosis is similar to that of ricin exposure—any biologic agent that can produce acute respiratory disease (eg, staphylococcal enterotoxin B, mycotoxins, anthrax, tularemia, plague). A toxin assay of implicated food and water, serum, sputum, or urine is required for a specific diagnosis [129]. The toxin also may be identified by ELISA of nasal swabs [121]. Serum antibodies may help confirm the diagnosis.

*Treatment.* Treatment is supportive in nature. Antibiotics are not recommended. A full recovery is expected after several weeks of incapacitation [14, 127–130]. Approximately 15% of patients require hospitalization, and a 5% fatality rate may be seen, particularly in patients of extreme ages. If death occurs, it is usually the result of respiratory failure [14].

*Infection control and prevention.* There is no potential for human-to-human spread [121], and secondary aerosolization is not considered a hazard [127]. No vaccines or antitoxins currently are available [14]. Soap and water decontamination is adequate [121].

*Staphylococcal enterotoxin B as a weapon.* The toxin is stable in aerosols and can produce severe incapacitating effects at low doses. Because of the short incubation period, a sudden cluster of cases in a localized area is more likely due to Staphylococcal enterotoxin B than any other biologic agent [121]. It is estimated that >80% of exposed individuals would be incapacitated [14].

*Alpha viruses*

*Virology.* Venezuelan, Eastern, and Western equine encephalitis viruses (VEE, EEE, WEE, respectively), members of the alpha virus genus of the family *Togaviridae*, are known to cause viral encephalitis in humans. These encephalitides are spread via a mosquito vector from a bird host in the case of EEE and WEE and a rodent host in the case of VEE. They are highly infectious via aerosol, with 10 to 100 organisms causing disease. Increasing virulence is seen from VEE, WEE, to EEE [131].

*Clinical presentation.* All human infections are symptomatic [105]. After inoculation via a mosquito bite, a febrile prodrome of 1 to 5 days follows and marks viral replication in the bone marrow and lymphoid tissue that results in lymphopenia [131]. A viral febrile syndrome that includes fever, headache, myalgia, photophobia, and vomiting begins [105]. Viremia ensues, which seeds the CNS. CNS signs and symptoms include meningismus, hyperactive and hypoactive reflexes, confusion, obtundation, dysphasia, seizures, paresis, ataxia, myoclonus, cranial nerve palsies, and even death [105,131]. All three viruses cause a leukopenia early, followed by a leukocytosis late. Serum aspartate aminotransferase levels are commonly elevated in VEE [105]. For patients with CNS involvement, a lumbar puncture is recommended. Patients with EEE commonly have an elevated opening pressure, and the CSF for all three viruses demonstrates a lymphocytic pleocytosis with cell counts up to $500 \times 10^6$/L [105] and an elevated protein [131]. EEE and WEE produce severe encephalitis; VEE in adults is a self-limited febrile illness. Approximately 4% of children with VEE, however, develop frank encephalitis with the potential for permanent neurologic sequelae and death [113].

*Diagnosis.* Virus isolation can be from a patient's serum, CSF, or throat washes. Generally hemagglutination-inhibiting ELISA and plaque-reduction neutralization antibodies are present by the second week of illness. Isolation of the virus or fourfold or greater titer rises in convalescent serum samples are diagnostic [105].

*Treatment.* The mortality rate for symptomatic EEE cases is between 50% and 75%, with most survivors developing permanent neurologic sequelae [113]. Treatment is mainly supportive and is aimed at specific symptoms.

*Infection control and prevention.* Human-to-human transmission is not thought to occur. A live-virus VEE vaccine, TC-83, has been used in laboratory workers for 40 years but remains investigational [113]. Inactivated vaccines for VEE, EEE, WEE are currently available under investigational new drug protocol [131] but are poorly immunogenic and require repeated immunization [132].

*Alpha viruses as a weapon.* VEE, although it causes less severe disease than EEE or WEE, is the one agent that has been weaponized because of its high disease-to-infection ratio (everyone infected develops a symptomatic illness), and VEE is highly infectious as an aerosol [113]. A large die-off of equine animals in an area should alert one to the possibility of an outbreak or bioterrorist event.

**Special circumstances**

We also must be ready to deal with the psychological casualties, persons directly involved in the attack and secondary casualties related to but peripheral to the event [40,133]. Decontamination of children poses special issues secondary to an unfamiliar environment, separation anxiety, and potential hypothermia [134,135].

**The role of oral and maxillofacial surgeons**

There are several roles that oral and maxillofacial surgeons would undertake. We would be at the forefront of facial trauma management because of injuries sustained in the attack from ballistic injury or motor vehicle collisions secondary to blast effect or collateral damage. Our medical and critical care training place us in a unique position to assist with the diagnosis of biologic agent infections and critical care interventions used to treat them. Our offices conceivably could be used as aid stations [136], postexposure prophylaxis dispensing sites, or even quarantine sites. As American Dental Association President T. Howard Jones stated, "When it comes to bioterrorism, there can be no spectators" [137]. It is recommended that all oral and maxillofacial surgeons become involved with their local hospital/community mass casualty response committees and take an active role in the preparation for a mass casualty bioterrorist event.

## Public health issues

Minimizing the risk of a bioterrorist event encompasses intelligence gathering, security, prevention (identifying potential primary sites of attacks), public awareness, disease surveillance, stockpiling of adequate resources, training of first responders/providers in disease recognition, biologic mass casualty hospital protocols and decontamination procedures, aggressive treatment of diseases with pharmacotherapeutic agents, isolation, quarantine and travel restrictions, and safe management of deceased victims. Disease surveillance encompasses the proper reporting of suspected disease outbreaks to the appropriate local and state health departments and the CDC. All of the diseases mentioned in this article are reportable diseases. The results of an American Academy of Dermatology survey are distressing. Only 11% of respondents believed that they were prepared to respond to a bioterrorist attack. Only 18% believed that they had received adequate training in the area of bioterrorism. Slightly more than half did not know where to report possible infections or whether they could recognize a bioterrorism-related disease. Worse, only 10% had a formal plan in place to deal with a bioterrorist event [138].

In a similar survey sent to emergency medicine residency directors, most believed that they were inadequately prepared to recognize and clinically manage casualties of a bioterrorist event. The survey also revealed a limited knowledge on how to access information regarding biologic weapons. Slightly more than half of the emergency medicine programs have biologic weapons training in their curriculum, but only 11% of these are field exercises [139]. The American Dental Association and American Dental Education Association reached a consensus that all dental students should be trained in a set of core competencies to enable them to respond to a bioterrorist attack, help contain the spread of disease, and participate in surveillance activities as directed by proper authorities [140]. The Israeli Defense Force Medical Corps has developed a 2-day core curriculum course for teaching the medical management of WMD casualties [141].

Planning for a bioterrorist attack should be at all levels: national (eg, Federal Emergency Management Agency, Department of Defense, CDC), state, local, hospital, and provider office [142]. At the hospital level, a WMD mass casualty response plan should be in place and rehearsed on a routine basis. This practice facilitates a smooth reaction/transition in a time of great stress during an actual event. Practice also helps reduce possible closure of facilities and staff injuries caused by contaminated casualties [143] and avoidance of duplication of treatment and the receipt of proper treatment once in the medical system [144]. On April 11, 1995, New York City conducted an unrehearsed, no-warning exercise that involved a simulated chemical attack on a subway station. First responders arrived at the scene to find "victims" lying unconscious on the mezzanine level of the station. Observing no smoke and unaware that "poison gas" was present, firefighters and police entered the station without proper protective gear and became casualties [142]. What is frightening is that in a survey of hospitals in Federal Emergency Management Agency region III (District of Columbia, Maryland, Virginia, West Virginia, Pennsylvania, and Delaware) before 2001, no respondents believed that their sites were fully prepared to handle a biologic event. Four rural hospitals had no decontamination plans [145].

The goals of decontamination are to prevent further agent absorption by patients and to protect health care providers and facilities from contamination [146]. There are questions concerning the legality of mass quarantines and travel restrictions after a bioterrorist attack that public health officials must work out. The economic and practical impact of a bioterrorist event would be enormous. On April 24, 1997, the B'nai B'rith Headquarters in Washington, DC received a package that contained a threatening note and a Petri dish labeled "*Anthracis yersinia*" that was leaking a red fluid. During the incident response, two city blocks were isolated, 109 building occupants were quarantined, and 30 people underwent decontamination. The incident turned out to be a hoax. News reports have quoted the estimated cost of one response at nearly $500,000 [147]. The anticipated cleanup from the 2001 anthrax attacks is estimated at more than $200 million [148].

## Future directions

Improved and more rapid diagnostic methods, new and better medications for treatment or prophylaxis, new vaccines, and antitoxin therapies are needed. Further research to define appropriate personal protective gear and decontamination procedures is required to improve our overall preparedness for a bioterrorist attack. On a global scale, we must look to the issue of how to reduce access to dangerous pathogens to prevent bioterrorism [149].

## Assessing future threats

According to Federal Bureau of Investigation testimony before the House Energy and Commerce Subcommittee on Oversight and Investigations in 1998, they investigated 181 cases of WMD, of which 112 involved bioterrorism. In 1999, the number of WMD cases increased to 267, with 187 involving bioterrorism. In 2000, the number of WMD cases was 257, of which 115 were bioterrorism related [150]. With the dissolution of the former Soviet Union, the potential exists for out-of-work scientists to sell their services to rogue states and terrorist organizations, helping them to develop biologic weapons [20]. Iraq, Iran, Syria, Libya, China, North Korea, Russia, Israel, Taiwan, Egypt, Viet Nam, Laos, Cuba, Bulgaria, and South Africa and possibly Sudan, India, and Pakistan are believed to possess or are pursuing offensive biologic weapons [151]. Threats may come from state-sponsored groups, independent or international terrorist groups, or lone individuals. These individuals or groups are "asymmetric threats" that attempt to circumvent the United States technologic and military superiority by attacking perceived weaknesses with new tactics, strategies, and weaponry. The September 11, 2001 attacks are a striking example of this asymmetric threat [7]. The ideal biologic weapons agent would display the following characteristics: (1) low infectious dose, (2) easy dissemination via an aerosol, (3) unavailability of an effective vaccine, (4) availability for procurement, (5) production in large quantities, (6) relative stability in the environment, and (7) previous use as weapons [12,33]. There is no reason to believe that the 2001 anthrax attacks will be an isolated incident. It is more likely that additional attacks will occur in the future [152].

## Further information

The following Websites are provided to the readership as access to further information via the Internet:

Centers for Disease Control and Prevention (www.bt.cdc.gov)
Association for Professionals in Infection Control and Epidemiology (www.apic.org)

University of Alabama at Birmingham Bioterrorism and Emerging Infections Education (www.bioterrorism.uab.edu)
Food and Drug Administration (www.fda.gov/oc/opacom/hottopics/bioterrorism.html)
American Medical Association (www.ama-assn.org/ama/pub/category/6206.html)
Johns Hopkins University Bloomberg School of Public Health (www.jhsph.edu)
Center for Biosecurity of the University of Pittsburgh Medical Center (www.upmc-biosecurity.org)
World Health Organization (www.who.int)

## Acknowledgments

The author wishes to acknowledge Samantha C. Bourgeois for her assistance in preparing the manuscript.

## References

[1] Huxsoll DL, Parrott CD, Patrick WC. Medicine in defense against biological warfare. JAMA 1989; 262(5):677–9.
[2] Klietmann WF, Ruoff KL. Bioterrorism: implications for the clinical microbiologist. Clin Microbiol Rev 2001;14(2):364–81.
[3] Henderson DA. Bioterrorism as a public health threat. Emerg Infect Dis 1998;4(3):488–92.
[4] Kortepeter M, Christopher G, Cieslak T, et al. Medical management of biologic casualties handbook. 4th edition. Fort Detrick, Frederick (MD): US Army Medical Research Institute of Infectious Diseases; 2001. p. 1–12.
[5] Jacobs MK. The history of biologic warfare and bioterrorism. Dermatol Clin 2004;22(3):231–46.
[6] Eitzen EM, Takafuji ET. Historical overview of biological warfare. In: Sidell FR, Takafuji EF, Franz DR, editors. Medical aspects of chemical and biological warfare. Washington, DC: Borden Institute; 1997. p. 415–23.
[7] Noah DL, Huebner KD, Darling RG, et al. The history and threat of biological warfare and terrorism. Emerg Med Clin North Am 2002;20(2):255–71.
[8] Robertson AG. From asps to allegations: biological warfare in history. Mil Med 1995;160(8):369–73.
[9] Derbes VJ. DeMussis and the great plague of 1348: a forgotten episode of bacteriological war. JAMA 1966;196(1):59–62.
[10] Smart JK. History of chemical and biological warfare: an American perspective. In: Sidell FR, Takafuji ET, Franz DR, editors. Medical aspects of chemical and

biological warfare. Washington, DC: Borden Institute; 1997. p. 9–86.

[11] Christopher GW, Cieslak TJ, Pavlin JA, et al. Biological warfare: a historical perspective. JAMA 1997; 278(5):412–7.

[12] Davis CJ. Nuclear blindness: an overview of the biological weapons programs of the former Soviet Union and Iraq. Emerg Infect Dis 1999;5(4):509–12.

[13] Olson KB. Aum Shinrikyo: once and future threat? Emerg Infect Dis 1999;5(4):513–6.

[14] Henghold WB. Other biologic toxin bioweapons: ricin, staphylococcal enterotoxin B, and trichothecene mycotoxins. Dermatol Clin 2004;22(3):257–62.

[15] Kadlec RP, Zelicoff AP, Vrtis AM. Biological weapons control: prospects and implications for the future. JAMA 1997;278(5):351–6.

[16] Alibek K. Biohazard. New York: Random House; 1999. p. 3–292.

[17] Rotz LD, Khan AS, Lillibridge SR, et al. Public health assessment of potential biological terrorism agents. Emerg Infect Dis 2002;8(2):225–30.

[18] Centers for Disease Control and Prevention. Biological and chemical terrorism: strategic plan for preparedness and response. Recommendations of the CDC strategic planning workgroup. MMWR Morb Mortal Wkly Rep 2000;49(No. RR-4):1–14.

[19] Breman JG, Henderson DA. Current concepts: diagnosis and management of smallpox. N Engl J Med 2002;346(17):1300–8.

[20] Henderson DA, Inglesby TV, Bartlett JG, et al. Smallpox as a biological weapon: medical and public health management. JAMA 1999;281(22):2127–37.

[21] O'Toole T. Smallpox: an attack scenario. Emerg Infect Dis 1999;5(4):540–6.

[22] Wehrle PF, Posch J, Richter KH, et al. An airborne outbreak of smallpox in a German hospital and its significance with respect to other recent outbreaks in Europe. Bull World Health Organ 1970;43(5): 669–79.

[23] Lupatkin H, Lupatkin JF, Rosenberg AD. Smallpox in the 21st century. Anesthesiol Clin North Am 2004; 22(3):541–61.

[24] Fenner F, Henderson DA, Arita I, et al. Smallpox and its eradication. Geneva (Switzerland): World Health Organization; 1988. p. iv.

[25] Harper GJ. Airborne micro-organisms: survival tests with four viruses. Am J Hyg 1961;59:479–86.

[26] Huq F. Effect of temperature and relative humidity on variola virus in crusts. Bull World Health Organ 1976;54(6):710–2.

[27] Slifka MK, Hanifin JM. Smallpox: the basics. Dematol Clin 2004;22(3):263–74.

[28] Tennyson HC, Mair EA. Smallpox: what every otolaryngologist should know. Otolaryngol Head Neck Surg 2004;130(3):323–33.

[29] Semba RD. The ocular complications of smallpox and smallpox immunization. Arch Ophthalmol 2003; 121(5):715–9.

[30] Wollenberg A, Engler R. Smallpox, vaccination and adverse reactions to smallpox vaccine. Curr Opin Allergy Clin Immunol 2004;4(4):271–5.

[31] Henderson DA. Smallpox: clinical and epidemiologic features. Emerg Infect Dis 1999;5(4):537–9.

[32] Centers for Disease Control and Prevention. Executive summary: smallpox response plan and guidelines. Available at: http://www.bt.cdc.gov/agent/smallpox/response-plan/index.asp. Accessed January 16, 2005.

[33] Darling RG, Catlett CL, Huebner KD, et al. Threats in bioterrorism I: CDC category A agents. Emerg Med Clin North Am 2002;20(2):273–309.

[34] Tom WL, Kenner JR, Friedlander SF. Smallpox: vaccine reactions and contraindications. Dermatol Clin 2004;22(3):275–89.

[35] Centers for Disease Control and Prevention. Recommendations for using smallpox vaccine in a pre-event vaccination program: supplemental recommendations of the Advisory Committee on Immunization Practices (ACIP) and the Healthcare Infection Control Practices Advisory Committee (HICPAC). Morb Mortal Wkly Rep MMWR 2003;52(No. RR-7):1–16.

[36] Centers for Disease Control and Prevention. Smallpox vaccination and adverse reactions: guidance for clinicians. MMWR Morb Mortal Wkly Rep 2003; 52(No. RR-4):1–28.

[37] Lane JM, Ruben FL, Neff JM, et al. Complications of smallpox vaccination, 1968: results of 10 statewide surveys. J Infect Dis 1970;122(4):303–9.

[38] Alibek K. Smallpox: a disease and a weapon. Int J Infect Dis 2004;8(Suppl 2):S3–8.

[39] Cieslak TJ, Christopher GW, Ottolini MG. Biological warfare and the skin II: viruses. Clin Dermatol 2002; 20(4):355–64.

[40] Benedek DM, Holloway HC, Becker SM. Emergency mental health management in bioterrorism events. Emerg Med Clin North Am 2002;20(2):393–407.

[41] Beasley A, Kenenally S, Mickel N, et al. Treating patients with smallpox in the operating room. AORN J 2004;80(4):681–9.

[42] Vukas A. Smallpox-induced scars: treatment by dermabrasion. Dermatologica 1974;148(3):175–8.

[43] Manchanda RL, Singh R, Keswani RK, et al. Dermabrasion in small-pox scars of the face. Br J Plast Surg 1967;20(4):436–40.

[44] Sternbach G. The history of anthrax. J Emerg Med 2003;24(4):463–7.

[45] Pile JC, Malone JD, Eitzen EM, et al. Anthrax as a potential biologic warfare agent. Arch Intern Med 1998;158(5):429–34.

[46] Shafazand S, Doyle R, Tuoss S, et al. Inhalational anthrax: epidemiology, diagnosis, and management. Chest 1999;116(5):1369–76.

[47] Inglesby TV, O'Toole T, Henderson DA, et al. Anthrax as a biological weapon, 2002. JAMA 2002;287(17):2236–52.

[48] Binkley CE, Cinti S, Simeone DM, et al. Bacillus anthracis as an agent of bioterrorism: a review emphasizing surgical treatment. Ann Surg 2002;236(1): 9–16.

[49] Bradley PJ, Ferlito A, Brandwein MS, et al. Anthrax: what should the otolaryngologist know? Acta Otolaryngol 2002;122(6):580–5.

[50] Shafazand S. When bioterrorism strikes: diagnosis and management of inhalational anthrax. Semin Respir Infect 2003;18(3):134–45.

[51] Spencer RC. Bacillus anthracis. J Clin Pathol 2003; 56(3):182–7.

[52] Wirtschafter A, Cherukuri S, Benninger MS. Anthrax: ENT manifestations and current concepts. Otolaryngol Head Neck Surg 2002;126(1):8–13.

[53] Soysal HG, Kirath H, Recep OF. Anthrax as the cause of preseptal cellulites and cicatricial ectropion. Acta Ophthalmol Scand 2001;79(2):208–9.

[54] Bekerecioglu M, Tercan M, Atik B, et al. Cutaneous anthrax of the eyelid. Ann Plast Surg 2001;46(4): 455–6.

[55] Faghihi G, Siadat AH. Cutaneous anthrax associated with facial palsy. Clin Exp Dermatol 2003;28(1): 92–3.

[56] Wenner KA, Kenner JR. Anthrax. Dermatol Clin 2004;22(3):247–56.

[57] Sirisanthana T, Navacharoen N, Tharavichitkul P, et al. Outbreak of oral-oropharyngeal anthrax: an unusual manifestation of human infection with Bacillus anthracis. Trop Med Hyg 1984;33(1):144–50.

[58] Navacharoen N, Sirisanthana T, Navacharoen W, et al. Oropharyngeal anthrax. J Laryngol Otol 1985; 99(12):1293–5.

[59] Quintiliani R, Quintiliani R. Inhalational anthrax and bioterrorism. Curr Opin Pulm Med 2003;9(3):221–6.

[60] George S, Mathai D, Balraj V, et al. An outbreak of anthrax meningoencephalitis. Trans R Soc Trop Med Hyg 1994;88(2):206–7.

[61] Nalin DR. Recognition and treatment of anthrax. JAMA 1999;282(17):1624–5.

[62] Sirisanthana T, Nelson KE, Ezzell JW, et al. Serological studies of patients with cutaneous and oral-oropharyngeal anthrax from northern Thailand. Am J Trop Med Hyg 1988;39(6):575–81.

[63] Cunha BA. Anthrax, tularemia, plague, Ebola or smallpox as agents of bioterrorism: recognition in the emergency room. Clin Microbiol Infect 2002;8(8): 489–503.

[64] Centers for Disease Control and Prevention. Update: interim recommendations for antimicrobial prophylaxis for children and breastfeeding mothers and treatment of children with anthrax. MMWR Morb Mortal Wkly Rep 2001;50(45):1014–6.

[65] Centers for Disease Control and Prevention. Update: investigation of anthrax associated with intentional exposure and interim public health guidelines, October 2001. MMWR Morb Mortal Wkly Rep 2001; 50(41):890–908.

[66] Bell DM, Kozarsky PE, Stephens DS. Conference summary: clinical issues in the prophylaxis, diagnosis, and treatment of anthrax. Emerg Infect Dis 2002;8(2):222–5.

[67] Cieslak TJ, Talbot TB, Harstein BH. Biological

warfare and the skin I: bacteria and toxins. Clin Dermatol 2002;20(4):346–54.

[68] McGovern TW, Norton SA. Recognition and management of anthrax. N Engl J Med 2002;346(12): 943–5.

[69] King P. Recognition and management of anthrax. N Engl J Med 2002;346(12):943–5.

[70] Swartz MN. Recognition and management of anthrax. N Engl J Med 2002;346(12):943–5.

[71] Aslan G, Terzioglu A. Surgical management of cutaneous anthrax. Ann Plast Surg 1998;41(5):468–70.

[72] Inglesby T, O'Toole T. Guidelines for treatment of anthrax. JAMA 2002;288(15):1849.

[73] Jernigan JA, Stephens DS, Ashford DA, et al. Bioterrorism-related inhalational anthrax: the first 10 cases reported in the United States. Emerg Infect Dis 2001;7(6):933–44.

[74] Cuneo BM. Inhalational anthrax. Respir Care Clin N Am 2004;10(1):75–82.

[75] Centers for Disease Control and Prevention. Update: investigation of bioterrorism-related anthrax and adverse events from antimicrobial prophylaxis. MMWR Morb Mortal Wkly Rep 2001;50(44):973–1000.

[76] Centers for Disease Control and Prevention. Use of anthrax vaccine in response to terrorism: supplemental recommendations of the advisory committee on immunization practices. MMWR Morb Mortal Wkly Rep 2002;51(45):1024–6.

[77] Centers for Disease Control and Prevention. Use of anthrax vaccine in the United States: recommendations of the advisory committee on immunization practices. MMWR Morb Mortal Wkly Rep 2000; 49(No. RR-15):1–17.

[78] World Health Organization. Health aspects of chemical and biological weapons. Geneva (Switzerland): World Health Organization; 1970. p. 97–9.

[79] Perry RD, Fetherston JD. Yersinia pestis: etiologic agent of plague. Clin Microbiol Rev 1997;10(1): 35–66.

[80] Lazarus AA, Decker CF. Plague. Respir Care Clin N Am 2004;10(1):83–98.

[81] Cobbs CG, Chansolme DH. Plague. Dermatol Clin 2004;22(3):303–12.

[82] Krishna G, Chitkara RK. Pneumonic plague. Semin Respir Infect 2003;18(3):159–67.

[83] Josko D. Yersinia pestis: still a plague in the 21st century. Clin Lab Sci 2004;17(1):25–9.

[84] Butler T. Plague. In: Strickland GT, editor. Hunter's tropical medicine. 6th edition. Philadelphia: WB Saunders; 1984. p. 340–8.

[85] Higgins JA, Ezzell J, Hinnebusch BJ, et al. 5′ Nuclease PCR assay to detect yersinia pestis. J Clin Microbiol 1998;36(8):2284–8.

[86] Chanteau S, Rahalison L, Ratsitorahina M, et al. Early diagnosis of bubonic plague using F1 antigen capture ELISA assay and rapid immunogold dipstick. Int J Med Microbiol 2000;290(3):279–83.

[87] Swartz MN. Yersinia, francisella, pasteurella and brucella. In: Davis B, Dulbecco R, Eisen HN, et al,

editors. Microbiology. 4<sup>th</sup> edition. Philadelphia: JB
Lippincott; 1990. p. 601–14.

[88] Inglesby TV, Dennis DT, Henderson DA, et al. Plague
as a biological weapon. JAMA 2000;283(17):2281–90.

[89] Dunbar EM. Botulism. J Infect 1990;20(1):1–3.

[90] Ting P, Freiman A. The story of clostridium
botulinum: from food poisoning to Botox. Clin
Med 2004;4(3):258–61.

[91] Erbguth FJ. Botulinum toxin: a historical note. Lancet
1998;351(9118):1820.

[92] Arnon SS, Schechter R, Inglesby TV, et al. Botulinum
toxin as a biological weapon. JAMA 2001;285(8):
1059–70.

[93] Centers for Disease Control and Prevention. Botulism
in the United States, 1899–1996: handbook for
epidemiologists, clinicians, and laboratory workers.
Atlanta (GA): Centers for Disease Control and
Prevention; 1998.

[94] Cherington M. Botulism: update and review. Semin
Neurol 2004;24(2):155–63.

[95] Arnon SS. Infant botulism. In: Feigen R, Cherry J,
editors. Textbook of pediatric infectious diseases.
Philadelphia: WB Saunders; 1992. p. 1095–102.

[96] Caya JG. Clostridium botulinum and the ophthalmologist: a review of botulism, including biological
warfare ramifications of botulinum toxin. Surv
Ophthalmol 2001;46(1):25–34.

[97] Robinson RF, Nahata MC. Management of botulism.
Ann Pharmacother 2003;37(1):127–31.

[98] Caya JG, Agni R, Miller JE. Clostridium botulinum
and the clinical laboratorian. Arch Pathol Lab Med
2004;128(6):653–62.

[99] Sotos JG. Botulinum toxin in biowarfare. JAMA
2001;285(21):2716.

[100] Rinaldo A, Bradley PJ, Ferlito A. Tularemia in
otolaryngology: a forgotten but not gone disease
and a possible sign of bio-terrorism. J Laryngol Otol
2004;118(4):257–9.

[101] Dennis DT, Inglesby TV, Henderson DA, et al.
Tularemia as a biological weapon: medical and public
health management. JAMA 2001;285(21):2763–73.

[102] Centers for Disease Control and Prevention. Tularemia: United States, 1990–2000. MMWR Morb
Mortal Wkly Rep 2002;51(9):181–204.

[103] Ellis J, Oyston PCF, Green M, et al. Tularemia. Clin
Microbiol Rev 2002;15(4):631–46.

[104] Jensen WA, Kirsch CM. Tularemia. Semin Respir
Infect 2003;18(3):146–58.

[105] Franz DR, Jahrling PB, Friedlander AM, et al.
Clinical recognition and management of patients
exposed to biological warfare agents. JAMA 1997;
278(5):399–411.

[106] Greenfield RA, Drevets DA, Machado LJ, et al. Bacterial pathogens as biological weapons and agents of
bioterrorism. Am J Med Sci 2002;323(6):299–315.

[107] Cronquist SD. Tularemia: the disease and the weapon.
Dermatol Clin 2004;22(3):313–20.

[108] Cerny Z. Skin manifestations of tularemia. Int J
Dermatol 1994;33(7):468–70.

[109] Jacobs RF. Tularemia. Adv Pediatr Infect Dis
1996;12:55–69.

[110] Croddy E, Krcalova S. Tularemia, biological warfare,
and the battle of Stalingrad (1942–1943). Mil Med
2001;166(10):837–8.

[111] Polesky A, Bhatia G. Ebola hemorrhagic fever in the
era of bioterrorism. Semin Respir Infect 2003;18(3):
206–15.

[112] Salvaggio MR, Baddley JW. Other viral bioweapons:
Ebola and Marburg hemorrhagic fever. Dermatol Clin
2004;22(3):291–302.

[113] Bronze MS, Huycke MM, Machado LJ, et al. Viral
agents as biological weapons and agents of bioterrorism. Am J Med Sci 2002;323(6):316–25.

[114] Sanchez A, Khan AS, Zaki SR, et al. Filoviridae:
Marburg and Ebola. In: Knipe DM, Howley PM,
Griffin DE, et al, editors. Fields virology. 4<sup>th</sup> edition.
Philadelphia: Lippincott; 2001. p. 1279–304.

[115] Slenczka WG. The Marburg outbreak of 1967 and
subsequent episodes. Curr Top Microbiol Immunol
1999;235:49–75.

[116] Madariaga MG, Rezai K, Trenholme GM, et al.
Q fever: a biological weapon in your backyard. Lancet Infect Dis 2003;3(11):709–21.

[117] Kagawa FT, Wehner JH, Mohindra V. Q fever as a
biological weapon. Semin Respir Infect 2003;18(3):
183–95.

[118] Wortmann G. Pulmonary manifestations of other
agents: brucella, Q fever, tularemia and smallpox.
Respir Care Clin N Am 2004;10(1):99–109.

[119] McCaul TF, Williams JC. Developmental cycle of
Coxiella burnetii: structure and morphogenesis of
vegetative and sporogenic differentiations. J Bacteriol
1981;147(3):1063–76.

[120] Ackland JR, Worswick DA, Marmion BP. Vaccine
prophylaxis of Q fever: a follow-up study of the
efficacy of Q-vax (CSL) 1985–1990. Med J Aust
1994;160(11):704–8.

[121] Moran GJ. Threats in bioterrorism II: CDC category
B and C agents. Emerg Med Clin North Am 2002;
20(2):311–30.

[122] Bellamy RJ, Freedman AR. Bioterrorism. Q J Med
2001;94(4):227–34.

[123] Sarinas PSA, Chitkara RK. Brucellosis. Semin Respir
Infect 2003;18(3):168–82.

[124] Centers for Disease Control and Prevention. Brucellosis. Available at: http://www.cdc.gov/ncidod/
dbmd/diseaseinfo/brucellosis_g.htm. Accessed January 22, 2005.

[125] Corbel MJ. Brucellosis: an overview. Emerg Infect
Dis 1997;3(2):213–21.

[126] Sauret JM, Vilissova N. Human brucellosis. J Am
Board Fam Pract 2002;15(5):401–6.

[127] Zapor M, Fishbain JT. Aerosolized biologic toxins as
agents of warfare and terrorism. Respir Care Clin N
Am 2004;10(1):111–22.

[128] Marks JD. Medical aspects of biologic toxins. Anesth
Clin North Am 2004;22(3):509–32.

[129] Greenfield RA, Brown BR, Hutchins JB, et al.

Microbiological, biological, and chemical weapons of warfare and terrorism. Am J Med Sci 2002; 323(6):326–40.

[130] Centers for Disease Control and Prevention. Investigation of a ricin-containing envelope at a postal facility: South Carolina, 2003. MMWR Morb Mortal Wkly Rep 2003;52(46):1129–31.

[131] Karwa M, Bronzert P, Kvetan V. Bioterrorism and critical care. Crit Care Clin North Am 2003;19(2): 279–313.

[132] White SM. Chemical and biological weapons: implications for anaesthesia and intensive care. Br J Anaesth 2002;89(2):306–24.

[133] Holloway HC, Norwood AE, Fullerton CS, et al. The threat of biological weapons: prophylaxis and mitigation of psychological and social consequences. JAMA 1997;278(5):425–7.

[134] Patt HA, Feigin RD. Diagnosis and management of suspected cases of bioterrorism: a pediatric perspective. Pediatrics 2002;109(4):985–92.

[135] Rotenberg JS, Burklow TR, Selanikio JS. Weapons of mass destruction: the decontamination of children. Pediatr Ann 2003;32(4):261–7.

[136] Weber CR. Dentistry's role in biodefense. Pa Dent J 2003;70(5):32–4.

[137] Miller DJ. Why should dentists be involved in bioterrorism? N Y State Dent J 2003;69(5):10–1.

[138] Carroll C, Balkrishnan R, Khanna V, et al. Bioterrorism preparedness in the dermatology community. Arch Dermatol 2003;139(12):1657–8.

[139] Pesik N, Keim M, Sampson TR. Do US emergency medicine residency programs provide adequate training for bioterrorism? Ann Emerg Med 1999;34(2): 173–6.

[140] Chmar JE, Ranney RR, Guay AH, et al. Incorporating bioterrorism training into dental education: report of ADA-ADEA terrorism and mass casualty curriculum development workshop. J Dent Edu 2004;68(11): 1196–9.

[141] Rubinshtein R, Robenshtok E, Eisenkraft A, et al.

Training Israeli medical personnel to treat casualties of nuclear, biologic and chemical warfare. Isr Med Assoc J 2002;4(7):545–8.

[142] Tucker JB. National health and medical services response to incidents of chemical and biological terrorism. JAMA 1997;278(5):362–8.

[143] Tan GA, Fitzgerald MC. Chemical-biological-radiological (CBR) response: a template for hospital emergency departments. Med J Aust 2002;177(4): 196–9.

[144] Keim M, Kaufmann AF. Principles for emergency response to bioterrorism. Ann Emerg Med 1999; 34(2):177–82.

[145] Treat KN, Williams JM, Furbee PM, et al. Hospital preparedness for weapons of mass destruction incidents: an initial assessment. Ann Emerg Med 2001;38(5):562–5.

[146] Lepler L, Lucci E. Responding to and managing casualties: detection, personal protection, and decontamination. Respir Care Clin N Am 2004;10(1):9–21.

[147] Anthrax cleanup set for NJ post office. Available at: www.cnn.com/2003/US/Northeast/10/21/anthrax. postoffice.ap. Accessed January 19, 2005.

[148] Dewan PK, Fry AM, Laserson K, et al. Inhalational anthrax outbreak among postal workers, Washington, DC, 2001. Emerg Infect Dis 2002;8(10):1066–72.

[149] Hamburg MA. Addressing bioterrorist threats: where do we go from here? Emerg Med Infect 1999;5(4): 564–5.

[150] Caruso JT. Testimony before the United States Senate Judiciary Subcommittee on Technology, Terrorism and Government Information. Available at: http:// www.fbi.gov/congress/congress01/caruso110601. htm. Accessed January 15, 2005.

[151] McGovern TW, Christopher GW, Eitzen E. Cutaneous manifestations of biological warfare and related threat agents. Arch Dermatol 1999;135(3):311–22.

[152] Lane HC, Fauci AS. Bioterrorism on the home front. JAMA 2001;286(20):2595–7.

ELSEVIER
SAUNDERS

Oral Maxillofacial Surg Clin N Am 17 (2005) 331–339

ORAL AND
MAXILLOFACIAL
SURGERY CLINICS
of North America

# Oral and Maxillofacial Injuries Experienced in Support of Operation Iraqi Freedom I and II

Michael J. Will, DDS, MD[a],[*], Tamer Goksel, DDS, MD[b],
Charles G. Stone, Jr, DDS[a], Michael J. Doherty, DDS[c]

[a]Department of Oral and Maxillofacial Surgery, Walter Reed Army Medical Center, 6900 Georgia Avenue NW,
Washington, DC 20307, USA
[b]Oral and Maxillofacial Surgery Service, Brooke Army Medical Center, Fort Sam Houston, TX 78234, USA
[c]Department of Oral and Maxillofacial Surgery, National Naval Medical Center, 8901 Wisconsin Avenue,
Bethesda, MD 20889, USA

Penetrating, perforating, and avulsive fragmentation injuries present a unique surgical challenge for oral and maxillofacial surgeons in the Iraqi theater of operation. Maxillofacial injuries encountered in Operation Iraqi Freedom (OIF) and Operation Enduring Freedom (OEF) have presented injury patterns not encountered previously in other large-scale armed conflicts. Current literature in the field of oral and maxillofacial surgery does not cover adequately the concerns that are inherent to care and treatment planning at an echelon III facility. This article addresses clinical and surgical practice guidelines that were developed by oral surgeons in theater and from feedback they received from higher echelons of care.

## Mechanisms of injury in the battlefield

Most (50%) combat casualties present to the combat support hospital with fragmentation injuries subsequent to improvised explosive devices and vehicle-borne improvised explosive devices. A significant number of other mechanisms of injury in the battlefield include rocket-propelled grenades, mortars (5%), grenades, gunshot (high and low velocity) projectiles (17%), and motor vehicle crashes.

## Radiographic evaluation of maxillofacial injuries

Not all maxillofacial injuries warrant CT evaluation. Mechanism of injury and the complexity of hard tissue involvement should direct this decision-making process. Panorex and the mandibular series (ie, right and left oblique, posteroanterior skull, lateral skull, Towne's view) are more than adequate in providing the information necessary in the diagnosis of mandibular fractures. Simple maxillary fractures can be diagnosed adequately with a facial series (ie, Caldwell's view, Water's view, lateral skull, submentalvertex view). Most battle casualties who present to the combat support hospital requiring maxillofacial consultation have fragmentation injuries. Maxillofacial fragmentation wounds of any size should be given high consideration for CT imaging. Some superficial fragmentation wounds can be localized readily with plain radiography (posteroanterior and lateral skull) and may not necessitate CT imaging. A concentrated physical examination, history of current illness, and mechanism of injury guide the practitioner to the appropriate imaging modality.

## Surgical airway

The oral surgeon in the theater of operation must assess early the need for a surgical airway. Although there is a fast turnaround time in transporting in-

* Corresponding author.
  *E-mail address:* Michael.will@na.amedd.army.mil
(M.J. Will).

1042-3699/05/$ – see front matter. Published by Elsevier Inc.
doi:10.1016/j.coms.2005.04.004

jured patients to a higher echelon of care, there seems to be a prolonged evacuation time during which patients are not observed closely. In the transportation process, these same patients are moved repeatedly and sometimes in close quarters. Any patient with an airway concern or any patient who is orally or nasally intubated with a high probability of endotracheal tube displacement should be considered for a tracheostomy in the controlled environment of the combat support hospital. Patients with panfacial trauma, severe midfacial fractures, prolonged intubation, or multiple systemic trauma that requires multiple trips to the operating room should undergo a tracheostomy before mobilization to the next echelon of care. All patients who present with emergent airways (cricothyrotomy) should have conversion of the cricothyrotomy to a tracheostomy before mobilization.

### Management of battlefield soft tissue injuries

Head and neck hemorrhage secondary to fragmentation wounds can be substantial. Immediately after the establishment of a secure airway and completion of the advanced trauma life support primary survey, local measures can be used to control bleeding. Packing with gauze, direct pressure, suture ligation, clamping, and electrocautery can be used to minimize blood loss. On admission to the emergency department and after initial evaluation, minor wound care can be addressed. Initial gross irrigation, débridement, packing, and dressing of wounds in the emergency treatment area can establish a better overall outcome, especially because gaining timely access to an operating room can vary tremendously (immediate to 12 hours), depending on urgency and surgical caseloads.

All fragmentation injuries should be considered contaminated. Prophylactic antibiotics are a must and should be initiated on admission. Tetanus prophylaxis should be instituted with all contaminated wounds. Thorough irrigation and débridement should be initiated as soon as possible. Meticulous débridement during the initial phase may avert unaesthetic results secondary to infections, foreign body granulomas, and hypertrophic scars. On extensive peppering of large surface areas of skin with dirt, gravel, grass, wood, and other organic materials, a pulsed lavage system with high volumes of sterile saline is effective. The high-volume lavage is then followed by meticulous débridement and gauze sponge wound cleansing with a dilute povidine-iodine solution. Deep lacerations should be explored thoroughly for nerve, ductal, and other vital structure damage. If the nature of the injury does not allow treatment of these vital structures, the structures should be identified and tagged for easier location in future reconstructive procedures.

Deep, penetrating wounds that are difficult to débride effectively should be packed with iodoform or regular gauze. One should place only a single dressing into these deep wounds to allow easy and complete removal at the next echelon of care. Superficial wounds and wounds that are effectively débrided should be closed primarily when possible. The best aesthetic results are achieved through the initial treatment phase. Wounds should be handled gently, soft tissues should be débrided conservatively, dead spaces should be obliterated with deep sutures, subcuticular sutures should reapproximate the dermis and allow a tension-free skin margin, and fine sutures should elevate the skin margins slightly. A detailed discharge or transfer summary should indicate wound care instructions and the specific date for suture removal.

### Management of facial burns

During OEF, the frequency of facial burns has been high because of the mechanisms of injury to which soldiers are exposed (eg, close range blast, improvised explosive devices, vehicle-borne improvised explosive devices, rocket-propelled grenades). The primary concern in the management of these patients is associated airway injuries. Immediate airway control with oral endotracheal intubation is essential. During direct laryngoscopy, one should inspect the upper airway for signs of edema and soot. Once the airway is secured, one can evaluate the orbits for compartment syndrome caused by the ensuing soft tissue edema. One should perform lateral canthotomy and cantholysis as indicated. Next, gently débride the face with sterile saline and gauze or sponge brushes. After thorough débridement, one should apply bacitracin ophthalmic ointment to the periorbital region and regular bacitracin ointment throughout. Avoid the use of silvadene on the face because of its caustic effects on the eyes. Significant soft tissue edema is expected in the initial postinjury period. The endotracheal tube should be secured to the upper dentition with 24 gauge circumdental wiring. This method of securing the endotracheal tube prevents umbilical tapes and other material from further injuring the soft tissues of the face and neck. The umbilical tape is better used to secure wire cutters around a patient's neck during transport.

## Management of mandibular fractures

At the echelon III level of care, treatment of the mandibular fracture is not required unless it has a direct bearing on the patency of the airway or the control of hemorrhage. Definitive reduction and fixation of a facial fracture are never life-saving measures, and the immediate treatment should be left to procedures that are vital in the resuscitation and stabilization of the injured patient. When time and space allow—and when in the best interest of the patient—some oral and maxillofacial surgical interventions may improve patient morbidity.

Many mandibular fractures seen in battlefield injuries present with associated avulsive soft tissue defects. The mechanism of injury from fragmentation wounds results in comminuted fractures, loss of intraoral soft tissues, and embedded tooth fragments throughout the soft tissues. Hard tissue débridement and periosteal stripping are kept to a minimum in this setting to allow the wounds to declare which tissues are vital and which are not. The objective is to maintain as much of the hard and soft tissues as possible. Obvious foreign bodies, root tips, minute alveolar chips, and fragments are removed, but all else is preserved for evaluation at the next level of care.

Treatment options of mandibular fractures in coalition forces and Iraqi civilians include (1) external fixation, using the Joe-Hall Morris appliance or the Hoffman II orthopedic wrist device, (2) arch bar stabilization with maxillomandibular fixation, and (3) skeletal fixation using surgical wires. Coalition forces are rapidly deployed (within 12 hours) to a higher echelon of care. Re-evaluation and treatment planning for definitive care are initiated within 7 to 10 days after injury at a major medical facility near the home of the service member. Enemy combatants fall into a different treatment category within the

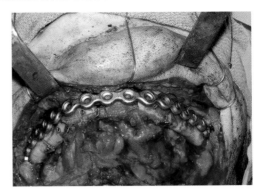

Fig. 2. Open reduction with internal fixation of mandibular fracture.

theater of operation. The Geneva Convention provisions require that definitive medical and surgical care be provided to enemy combatants once captured. The treatment plan for enemy combatants is established on initial evaluation. The surgical treatments can be sequenced to provide the patient the standard of care that has been established in Iraq. Depending on the degree of injury, mandibular fractures in detainees can be treated as outlined previously for coalition forces or can be treated using open reduction internal fixation techniques.

External pin fixation of comminuted fractures of the facial skeleton using the Hoffman II wrist external fixation kit has proved to be an expedient method of treating ballistic maxillofacial comminuted injuries (Fig. 1). The indications for open reduction and internal fixation of these injuries in the battlefield environment are limited because of limited operating room time, a high volume of casualties, and limited hospital beds (Fig. 2). This technique is faster than traditional biphasic external fixation and is just as effective. The kit is readily available, expedient, and disposable and offers the same benefits of immobilization of fractures, wound management, and delayed primary reconstruction at medical centers in the continental United States. The use of primary external fixation followed by delayed primary reconstruction results in decreased morbidity compared with primary reconstruction with bone plates and screws in the austere combat environment.

## Management of maxillary fractures

As with mandibular fractures, treatment of maxillary fractures is not required unless it has a direct bearing on the patency of the airway or in the control of hemorrhage. Severe maxillary and bilateral para-

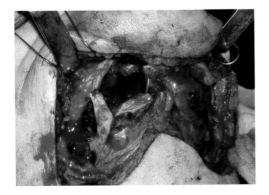

Fig. 1. Blast-related comminuted mandibular fracture.

nasal sinus injuries may necessitate a tracheostomy before patient transportation. The tracheostomy alleviates the need for nasal and oral manipulation and provides better nasal and oral hygiene for the patient. Tracheostomy access also provides better pulmonary toiletry for the patient.

In severe midface fractures, the primary concern is maintaining a patent airway. Fragmentation injuries to the midface usually result in an oral cavity that is filled with secretions, blood, and debris that consists of teeth, bone, and foreign body fragments. The oral cavity should be evaluated thoroughly, secretions and debris should be removed, and gauze packing should be inserted as needed for hemostasis. Initial examination in the emergency department also should rule out cerebrospinal fluid otorrhea and rhinorrhea, especially if there is evidence of basilar skull fracture. Any such evidence mandates a prompt consultation with a neurosurgeon.

Ocular injuries commonly are associated with midfacial trauma. Initial examination in the emergency department should include evaluation of both orbits for compartment syndrome, which results from intraorbital or retrobulbar hemorrhage. Even if there is a low level of suspicion, a lateral canthotomy and cantholysis should be initiated. All facial fractures that involve the orbits require an ophthalmologic consultation (Figs. 3, 4).

A nasal speculum examination in midface injuries can assist in the detection of septal hematomas. This condition requires prompt surgical drainage to prevent secondary infections and septal necrosis that results in a septal perforation. Merocel sponge packing after surgical drainage prevents reaccumulation of blood. It is imperative that the sponge packing

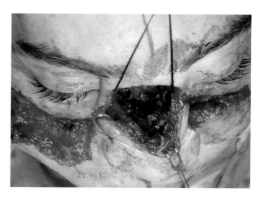

Fig. 4. Naso-orbital-ethmoid penetrating trauma.

be removed at 72 hours or earlier to prevent sinus infections or toxic shock.

Coalition forces who sustain LeFort-type fractures, including palatal fractures, are treated with maxillomandibular fixation if adequate intercuspation of the remaining dentition is achieved. Other options include external fixation using the Hoffman II wrist appliance in the severely comminuted midface and skeletal fixation using surgical wires. Detainees who sustain midface fractures can be treated as mentioned previously or with rigid fixation using a craniofacial plating system.

Zygomaticomaxillary complex fractures are second only to nasal fractures in their frequency in facial trauma. Treatment of these fractures is nonurgent, and care can be deferred to the next higher echelon with military patients or to the Iraqi civilian hospital system with host nationals. Detainees who require definitive care can undergo the standard approaches to reduce the fractures. Priority in care is provided to detainees who have functional deficits from their injuries. Some common deficits noted with zygomaticomaxillary complex fractures include trismus caused by possible temporalis muscle impingement and diplopia secondary to entrapment of extraocular muscles. Facial injuries without functional deficits and injuries that result only in cosmetic deformities are treated as time and space allows.

The use of craniofacial plating should be avoided in contaminated wounds and wounds with large soft tissue defects. Most coalition forces are transferred out of the theater within 24 to 72 hours, so rigid fixation with plating should be deferred until the patient is seen at a US military treatment facility and the tissues of the wound have declared their vitality. Use of internal rigid fixation (plates and screws) in fragmentation injuries to the face has resulted in high wound dehiscence and infection rates during OIF II. In our experience, thorough irrigation and

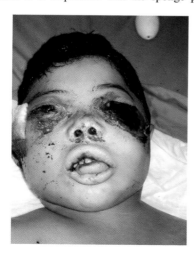

Fig. 3. Penetrating midface and orbital trauma.

débridement, conservative tissue management, and fracture stabilization with external fixation techniques have been most successful. Once the wound declares itself, secondary procedures using open reduction internal fixation have a much higher success rate.

## Management of otologic disorders

Troops who operate in a combat theater are subject to a wide variety of noise pollution. Hearing loss has been a common complaint of troops redeploying to the United States after service in OIF. It is well documented that hearing loss can affect a soldier's ability to perform the mission. Combat soldiers with hearing loss may not be able to perform their primary mission, and they may put themselves and others at risk. All soldiers should be advised to wear appropriate hearing protection when necessary. Soldiers with complaints of hearing loss should be tested audiometrically. Ideally, a previous audiogram should be available for comparison. If they have been wearing hearing protection and have sustained significant hearing loss (one "H" level or more), they should be removed from the high noise environment for 2 to 3 weeks. The audiogram should be repeated, and if the hearing loss has improved, soldiers may return to duty with the proper hearing protection. If the hearing loss has not improved, consideration must be given to reassigning soldiers to different duties or evacuating them from the theater.

Hearing loss from impulse noise (eg, explosions, gunshots) should be evaluated by audiologic testing at 24 to 72 hours after injury when possible. There is an initial deterioration of hearing after a blast, which makes an immediate audiogram less valuable as a baseline study. The hearing loss from impulse noise may be temporary or permanent. The reparative process for acute acoustic trauma lasts a minimum of 10 days and may take up to several weeks. Medical treatment is still experimental. There is no proven benefit to steroids. There is some evidence that high doses of vitamin $B_{12}$, cochlear ATP, or antioxidant therapy may be beneficial, but conclusive proof is still pending. Hearing loss that remains at 1 month after injury is considered to be permanent. At the 1-month mark, a decision can be made as to whether a soldier is capable of safely performing his or her duties. Asymmetric hearing loss not related to acoustic trauma should be evaluated to rule out acoustic neuroma. The screening test of choice is contrast MRI.

Approximately 80% of tympanic membrane perforations from acoustic trauma heal spontaneously. The extent of the perforation is estimated by the tympanic membrane surface area involved. Perforations heal at a rate of 10% per month. Ears with perforated tympanic membranes should be kept dry. In the presence of drainage, infection, or debris in the canal, a patient should be placed on antibiotic drops. If available, an otolaryngologist should evaluate the perforation. The canal can be cleaned, inverted mucosal edges can be unrolled, and a paper patch may be applied to aid in healing and protecting the middle ear. Surgical repair of residual perforations can be accomplished anywhere from 3 to 10 months. Tympanic membrane perforations are almost always associated with a hearing loss, so soldiers should be evaluated on their ability to perform their mission.

Tinnitus is commonly seen with sensorineural hearing loss. Patients should be advised to avoid the use of aspirin. The tinnitus may resolve as the hearing loss improves. New onset of tinnitus not associated with a progressive symmetric sensorineural hearing loss or with asymmetric acute acoustic trauma requires further investigation.

Vertigo may result from various conditions, including viral infections, otologic disorders (eg, Meniere's disease), head trauma, and brain tumors. On rare occasions, vertigo may be associated with severe acoustic trauma. Initially, vertigo may be managed with symptomatic treatments. Labyrinthine suppressants, such as meclizine or valium, may be used. Vertigo that persists beyond 2 weeks requires further evaluation and consultation with an otolaryngologist.

## Initial management: days 3 to 10

On average, soldiers injured in OIF/OEF arrive at a continental United States military treatment facility within 72 to 96 hours after injury. According to the sustained injuries, the soldiers typically arrive intubated and sedated. Upon arrival, the soldiers are triaged and admitted to the appropriate service for care and specialty consultations as needed (Fig. 5). Accompanying discharge summaries are reviewed as an aid to identify rapidly any acute issues and to guide ordering of additional studies.

Patients with oral or maxillofacial injuries are assessed clinically and radiographically as indicated. The clinical evaluation is approached in a standard head-to-toe fashion starting with the scalp and proceeding inferiorly to the clavicles. The soft tissue is evaluated for burns, lacerations, contusions, abrasions, pressure sores, and any other abnormalities. Attention is then directed to the bony skeleton, where manual palpation of the skeleton is performed extraorally and intraorally to feel for any steps or

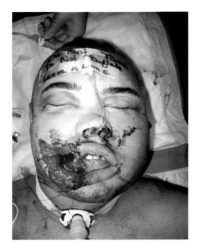

Fig. 5. Initial presentation at a higher echelon of care.

crepitus. A neurologic evaluation is performed to assess cranial nerve function, with deficits noted. A general ophthalmologic examination is performed in patients who are able to respond and follow commands. The external auditory canals and tympanic membranes are examined to assess for evidence of hemorrhage, laceration, edema, or tympanic membrane perforations. An intranasal evaluation is performed to evaluate septal position and hematoma. After a thorough clinical evaluation, patients with any level of suspicion for facial fractures receive a fine-cut (1.25-mm) CT scan without contrast in an axial and coronal view. The CT scans are then reviewed and diagnoses are rendered.

For patients with maxillofacial injuries that require intervention, a treatment plan is then formulated. Secondary to multisystemic trauma (notably orthopedic injuries and the need for multiple washouts), coordination with other services is necessary to optimize the patient's medical status and decrease overall anesthetic exposure time. Many patients also have associated intracranial injuries and may or may not be status post craniotomies, so neurosurgical clearance is often a factor in surgical planning. Cervical spine clearance is obtained unless specific documentation as to clearance at a previous echelon of care is provided.

## Treatment planning

In patients who require surgical intervention, airway management is the first consideration. Although many patients have tracheostomies in place, a decision must be made as to patients who remain

intubated. As in the civilian setting, if a prolonged intubation is anticipated, a prophylactic tracheostomy should be performed. Otherwise, the endotracheal tube is secured, used for the operating room, and the patient is extubated in the immediate postoperative period. One caveat involves the need for maxillomandibular fixation in relation to the airway. If extubation is planned in the immediate postoperative phase, a submental intubation may be performed, which may require replacing the endotracheal tube or an armored tube to ease in passage through the submental region. For patients with anticipated long intensive care unit stays secondary to respiratory issues or multiple surgeries, a tracheostomy is performed (Fig. 6).

In patients who have complex maxillofacial trauma, we routinely obtain a three-dimensional computerized reconstruction and a stereolithic model (Fig. 7). We have found these tools to be invaluable in treatment planning and preoperative model surgery. With such planning and pre-bending of plates, operating time is reduced. This is important in the patient who has multisystemic trauma and who is undergoing numerous procedures by multiple services. Decreasing the anesthetic exposure time is critical, notably with neurosurgical issues that face many of the patients.

As with all cases of trauma, treatment goals are to address hard and soft tissue injuries within the first 10 days, with an emphasis on initial management of soft tissue injuries caused by the large avulsive nature of the injury pattern. Current trauma texts regarding soft tissue injuries to the maxillofacial region place emphasis on early débridement and primary closure of such wounds. Through early fixation of fractures and replacement of the soft tissues, excellent functional and aesthetic results have been achieved in patients treated in our trauma centers. Most civilian trauma center patients, including most patients in-

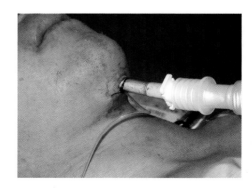

Fig. 6. Submental intubation.

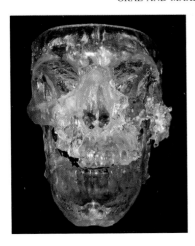

Fig. 7. Stereolithographic 3-D facial model.

volved in motor vehicle accidents, have maxillofacial injuries as a result of a low-energy phenomenon. Patients injured in OIF/OEF are unique. With high-velocity ballistic or avulsive injuries, the tissue damage, including the vasculature, extends beyond the grossly visible damage. Extensive literature exists in the orthopedic realm as to the importance of serial débridement and meticulous soft tissue management as keys to decreasing morbidity in such injuries. Many researchers have argued that because of the high vascularity of the maxillofacial region compared with long bones, similar assumptions should not be applied to the head and neck region. Our experience lends support to that of our colleagues in the orthopedic realm.

In our experience with soldiers who have taken part in OIF, serial débridement is indicated for three main reasons. The first reason involves the cavitation effect of a high-energy impact on tissues. Clark and colleagues [1] suggest that with this type of injury, "sufficient soft tissue damage occurs that an evolving pattern of tissue loss is observed." In dealing with patients who had early primary closure and subsequent wound "infection," exploration of such wounds revealed dusky and necrotic tissues in the normal pattern of wound breakdown rather than a grossly obvious infectious process.

The second factor involved with patients who have returned from OIF is their geographic location at time of injury. Trauma experienced in war or as a result of terrorist-related activities often involves the patient being in an austere environment for a period of time before transfer. Such patients have contaminated or even dirty wounds, which further supports the need for serial débridement. Patients are compromised secondary to nutritional status, sleep deprivation, and a high stress environment.

Finally, wound care during transport to a higher echelon of care is less than optimal or nonexistent; packings placed in theater are not removed until a patient's return to the United States, which leaves an ideal environment for bacterial growth. In patients who present with extensive packing, it should be obvious that the area is seeded and initial primary closure is contraindicated.

Many patients undergo irrigation and débridement in theater (Fig. 8). Secondary to the austere environment and the contaminated nature of an improvised explosive device, it has been our experience that patients with significant soft tissue injuries have a high rate of infection and wound breakdown despite the use of broad-spectrum antibiotics while en route to the United States. Our experience has altered our management in the past several years. Initially, in the spring of 2003, our approach was to treat maxillofacial injuries as would a civilian trauma center. Wounds were addressed within the first 48 hours of arrival (4 days after injury) with aggressive irrigation and débridement and primary closure. The immediate postoperative course was unremarkable until approximately day 5, when patients often declared an infection systemically or locally. Upon return to the operating room, no gross infections were observed. Although limited by the long-term antibiotic therapy, cultures were inconclusive. Our experience has demonstrated that wounds created by high-velocity weapons with multiple fragments declare themselves after the initial trauma phase and present as local fat necrosis, dusky wound margins, and local tissue dieback with extension into subcutaneous planes.

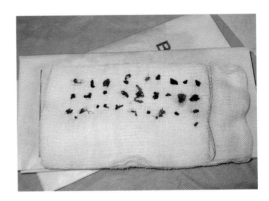

Fig. 8. Debris removed during serial débridement.

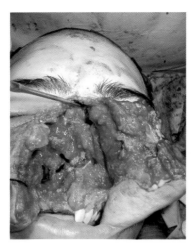

Fig. 9. Naso-orbital-ethmoid and orbital repair performed during third (and final) washout. Definitive flap reconstruction is deferred for secondary phase of treatment.

Based on our experience, we have altered our algorithm to coincide with recommendations from Clark and colleagues [1]. Patients with soft tissue injuries are routinely taken to the operating room for a thorough examination of all injured sites and débridement, including a pulsavac lavage. Primary closure is performed on wounds with no gross contamination and limited deep extension of the wound. Otherwise, after aggressive irrigation, the wound is packed with bacitracin-coated iodoform gauze and the wound margins are grossly reapproximated. Patients are then scheduled for serial washouts with definitive closure performed as warranted. We emphasize that initial attempts at primary closure using advancement or rotational flaps should be postponed until there is minimal risk for infection or additional tissue loss.

After initial wound healing, much emphasis is placed on efforts to alleviate initial scar contracture. Although this topic is discussed elsewhere, we cannot underestimate the devastating nature of scar contracture from high-velocity and avulsive injuries. Other factors, such as hemearthrosis/fibrous ankylosis of the joints and fibrosis of the muscles of mastication secondary to limited physical therapy caused by grave medical status and intensive care unit admissions, have led to much difficulty with long-term reconstruction. Kawaguchi and colleagues [2] reported that as much as 33% of patients who undergo postfrontotemporal procedures suffer from temporalis fibrosis and decreased maximal incisal opening. We have been aggressive with initial physical therapy, scar massage, and early steroid injections

and have seen significant improvement with short-term outcomes.

In contrast to the more classic approach of treating the bony skeleton first or in conjunction with the soft tissue, we have placed emphasis on soft tissue débridement with definitive fixation of the bony skeleton once edema resolves. Reconstructive efforts also are performed once initial wound healing has taken place; bone grafting, alloplastic implants, fat transfer, soft tissue recontouring, vestibulotplasty, and dental implants are deferred for several months to allow adequate healing and optimize reconstruction efforts.

Specific bony injuries from high-energy devices do require early intervention. We have opted to address naso-orbital-ethmoid fractures, canthal ligament resuspension, and reconstruction of orbital architecture early, often in conjunction with initial soft tissue washout procedures (Fig. 9). Extensive open reduction with internal fixation procedures are delayed until completion of serial washouts. With bony injuries that are blunter in nature and with minimal soft tissue destruction, standard panfacial sequencing and repair apply.

## References

[1] Clark N, Birely B, Manson PN, et al. High-energy ballistic and avulsive facial injuries: classification, patterns, and an algorithm for primary reconstruction. Plast Reconstr Surg 1996;98:583–601.
[2] Kawaguchi M, Sakamoto T, Furuya H, et al. Pseudoankylosis of the mandible after supratentorial craniotomy. Anesth Analg 1996;86:731–4.

## Further readings

Abubaker OA, Benson KJ. Oral and maxillofacial surgery secrets. Philadelphia: Hanley & Belfus; 2001.

Al-Qurainy A, Stassen LA, Dutton GN. The characteristics of midfacial fractures and the association with ocular injury: a prospective study. Br J Oral Maxillofac Surg 1991;29: 291–301.

Banks P. Killey's fractures of the mandible. 3rd edition. Bristol (UK): John Wright & Sons Ltd.; 1985.

Banks P. Killey's fractures of the middle third of the facial skeleton. 4th edition. Bristol (UK): John Wright & Sons Ltd.; Parr R, LeBanc J. Use of the Hoffman II wrist external fixation kit. 1984.

Booth PW. Maxillofacial trauma and esthetic facial reconstruction. New York: Churchill-Livingstone; 2003.

Casler J. Recommendations for treatment of otologic disorders. 2004

Fonseca R, editor. Oral and maxillofacial surgery. Philadelphia: WB Saunders; 2000.

Fonseca RJ, Walker RV, Betts NJ, et al. Oral and maxillofacial trauma. 2nd edition. Philadelphia: WB Saunders; 1997.

French B, Tornetta P. High-energy tibial shaft fractures. Orthop Clin North Am 2002;33:211–30.

Papel ID, Frodel J, Holt RG, et al. Facial plastic and reconstructive surgery. 2nd edition. New York: Thieme Medical Publishers; 2002.

ELSEVIER
SAUNDERS

Oral Maxillofacial Surg Clin N Am 17 (2005) 341 – 355

ORAL AND
MAXILLOFACIAL
SURGERY CLINICS
of North America

# Maxillofacial Trauma Treatment Protocol

David B. Powers, DMD, MD[a],*, Michael J. Will, DDS, MD[b],
Sidney L. Bourgeois, Jr, DDS[c], Holly D. Hatt, DMD, MD[d]

[a]*Department of Oral and Maxillofacial Surgery, Wilford Hall United States Air Force Medical Center, Lackland Air Force Base,
2200 Bergquist Drive, Suite 1, San Antonio, TX 78236-9908, USA*
[b]*Department of Oral and Maxillofacial Surgery, Walter Reed Army Medical Center, Washington, DC 20327, USA*
[c]*Department of Oral and Maxillofacial Surgery, National Naval Medical Center, Bethesda, MD 20889, USA*
[d]*Department of Oral and Maxillofacial Surgery, National Naval Medical Center, San Diego, CA 92127, USA*

In the early days of World War I, a young surgeon from New Zealand stationed in Aldershot, England was inundated by horrendous wounds to the head and neck of soldiers returning from the front lines. Because of advances in ballistics and weaponry, coupled with the fact that trench warfare necessitated the soldiers to place their maxillofacial region at great risk to monitor the status of the enemy, this surgeon was faced with injuries never before encountered. His name was Harold Delf Gillies, and his contributions to the medical community are universally accepted as the initiation of the discipline of plastic and reconstructive surgery [1,2]. Hippocrates once famously told his students, "War is the only proper school for surgeons." Unfortunately, the experiences undergone since September 11, 2001 have provided a whole generation of military surgeons the opportunity to treat a new type of injury pattern never before seen [3]. Improved body armor, which allows soldiers to survive wounds that would have been fatal 2 to 3 years earlier, and the catastrophic and new injury patterns sustained by improvised explosive devices (IEDs)

have forced military surgeons to reinvent how we treat maxillofacial trauma patients, much like the experiences that faced Sir Harold Gillies. Unfortunately, the Israeli experience shows us that terrorists possibly could use the same tactics as the Iraqi insurgents and expose the American populace to IEDs.

Before September 11, 2001, the protocol designed by Robertson and Manson served as an excellent framework for the management of high-energy ballistic injuries to the maxillofacial region [4]. The complex nature of the wounds caused by IEDs and newer ballistics has rendered some portions of their treatment plan ineffective and prone to secondary infection. IEDs are packed with dirt, glass, rocks, metal, bones from dead humans or animals, and other body parts if detonated by suicide bombers. If this technique of terrorism is used in the United States, civilian providers will be faced with the same difficulties previously faced by the military. The challenge was to develop a system that could be used for conventional ballistic injuries and injuries that result from IEDs. A new protocol has been developed that serves as the current treatment regimen used by the oral and maxillofacial surgery departments at Wilford Hall USAF Medical Center, the National Naval Medical Center–Bethesda, Walter Reed Army Medical Center, and the National Naval Medical Center–San Diego. In this article we present our treatment algorithm for ballistic maxillofacial trauma based on the surgical experiences gained by performing 329 procedures on 109 patients since September 2001 (Box 1).

The views presented in this article reflect those of the authors and do not represent the official policies of the United States Air Force, the United States Army, the United States Navy, the Department of Defense, or any branches of the United States government.
* Corresponding author.
*E-mail address:* David.Powers@Lackland.af.mil (D.B. Powers).

**Box 1. Treatment protocol for maxillofacial injuries**

1. Stabilize patient
2. Identify injuries
3. Obtain radiographic studies and stereolithographic models
4. Initiate consultations (eg, psychiatry, physical therapy, speech therapy)
5. Initiate cultures/sensitivities (infectious disease consultations)
6. Undertake serial débridement (days 3 – 10) to remove necrotic tissues
7. Stabilize hard tissue base to support soft tissue envelope and prevent scar contracture before primary reconstruction
8. Conduct comprehensive review of stereolithographic models and radiographs and determination of treatment goals
9. Replace missing soft tissue component (if necessary)
10. Perform primary reconstruction and fracture management
11. Incorporate aggressive physical/occupational therapy
12. Perform secondary reconstruction (eg, implants, vestibuloplasty)
13. Perform tertiary reconstruction (eg, cosmetic issues, scar revisions)

### Stabilization of the patient

Although this should be intuitive, in a mass casualty or acute trauma situation the basics of medical care should be emphasized, because these actions undoubtedly will save lives. Securing the airway by whatever means necessary, including endotracheal intubation or surgical airway, should be performed immediately if there is any doubt about future stability of the patient. A true disaster scenario easily could overwhelm the ability of a medical care facility to monitor the condition of victims with possible or suspected future airway compromise. Bleeding should be controlled and volume expansion should be accomplished to maintain perfusion of the vital organs by blood transfusion, blood substitutes,

colloids, or crystalloids as indicated. Identification of potentially fatal situations, such as tension pneumothorax, cardiac tamponade, intraperitoneal hemorrhage, or intracranial hemorrhage, should be accomplished as soon as possible.

### Identification of injuries

After initial stabilization of a patient, a thorough examination should be performed to document all injuries. If a patient is comatose or intubated or the evaluation is otherwise compromised, care should be taken to note clearly the limitations of the examination and the reasons for the difficulty. Detailed documentation of all injuries is necessary to coordinate the sequence of treatment with all respective surgical services (Figs. 1 and 2). Any opportunity to limit exposure to general anesthesia should be taken, as long as combined procedures do not affect the outcome of planned surgical interventions. Physical examination, radiographic studies, and laboratory tests are necessary components to identify correctly all potential injuries.

### Obtaining radiographic studies and stereolithographic models

Adequate radiographs are essential for diagnosis of and treatment planning for complex maxillofacial

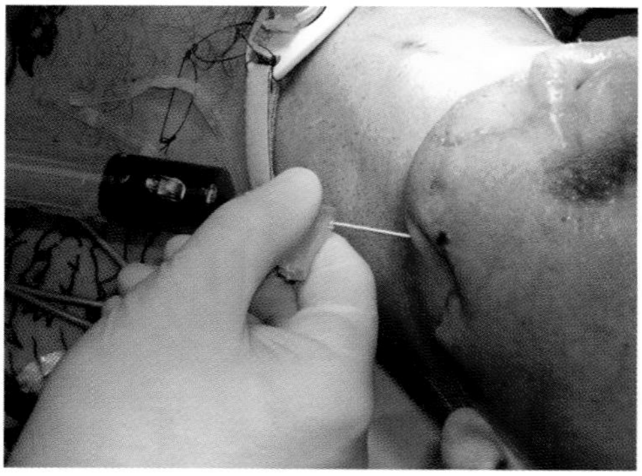

Fig. 1. Drainage of left facial swelling. After fluid was sent to laboratory for evaluation, amylase level was noted to be in excess of 3000, which is consistent with obstructed parotid gland secondary to transection of Stenson's duct from shrapnel.

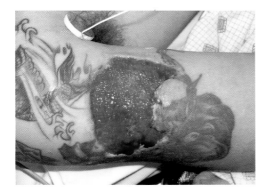

Fig. 2. Shrapnel injury to right upper extremity.

trauma. Modern radiographic techniques allow for three-dimensional visualization of the skeleton, help identify foreign bodies, and evaluate displaced fracture segments. CT scans should be the minimum information obtained before surgery (Fig. 3). The current CT scanner at Wilford Hall Medical Center is the GE Lightspeed 16 (GE Health Care, Chalfont St. Giles, United Kingdom), which allows rapid assimilation of data and manipulation of conventional coronal and axial cuts to three-dimensional images via use of the GE Advantage Workstation AW 4.1 (GE Health Care; Chalfont St. Giles, United Kingdom) (Fig. 4).

It is our opinion that complex panfacial trauma, such as the injuries seen during Operations Iraqi Freedom (OIF) and Enduring Freedom (OEF), absolutely require the fabrication of stereolithographic (SL) models to plan treatment adequately and determine sequencing of fracture repair. The use of SL models allows preadaptation of surgical plates to obtain proper soft tissue projection and support that otherwise would not be possible to the degree of accuracy obtained by this technique (Fig. 5). SL modeling has the advantage of allowing custom implant fabrication to support the soft tissue envelope when the bony architecture is lost or irreversibly misshapen. This has the advantage of reproducing a patient's preoperative soft tissue profile as close as possible to the preinjured state. Currently, Wilford Hall Medical Center transfers conventional CT data via the Materialise Mimics software program (Materialise, Leuven, Belgium) for model fabrication by the Viper SLA (3D Systems, Valencia, California). Depending on the size of the image being manufactured, most SL models can be completed by the Viper SLA within 6 to 24 hours. This relatively rapid turnaround time does not impact patient care and is essential in our experience for obtaining the best possible result while actually decreasing surgical time [5].

## Early initiation of consultations

Returning casualties from a war zone have many needs that must be addressed in concert to treat the entire patient. Not only is the treatment of a patient's wounds of paramount importance but also are the treatment of a patient's psychological status, facilitation of speech and nutrition in maxillofacial injuries, management of centrally mediated pain syndromes, and identification, evaluation, and involvement of a patient's family or peer support system. This section attempts to identify consultants who may be deemed integral in the treatment of returning casualties with war injuries.

### Infectious disease

The importance of this consultation cannot be overemphasized. Patients returning from OIF/OEF are well documented to be colonized by *Acinetobacter baumannii* [6]. The nature of war injuries also provides an environment for the gross contamination of wounds by staphylococci, enterococci, *Klebsiella,* and *Clostridium perfringens* and *Clostridium tetani.* Further discussions of the infectious disease consultation and the use of culture and sensitivity testing to facilitate treatment are presented in the following section.

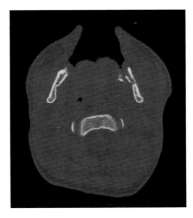

Fig. 3. Conventional CT scan indicates loss of soft tissue and anterior mandible extending bilaterally from the angle to angle.

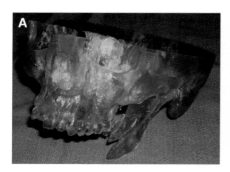
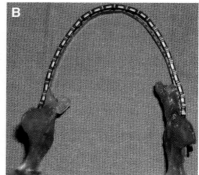

Fig. 4. (*A*) Stereolithography model of case presented in Fig. 3. (*B*) Model used as template for prebending of reconstruction bar.

## Psychiatry consultations

Injured patients who return from a war zone may present with a host of psychiatric challenges, all of which must be addressed for appropriate treatment of the patient. These stressors include unrecognized combat stress, depression related to an injury, and guilt related to leaving fellow unit members or surviving. Facial appearance has been found to be an important variable in how patients are perceived by others, and maxillofacial injury patients must develop the additional coping skills throughout their treatment to improve their self-esteem and ability to continue with reconstructive surgery.

## Nutrition and speech therapy consultations

Avulsive injuries to the maxillofacial region remove vital structures for phonation, mastication, and deglutition, and even if many of these structures are salvaged or reconstructed, injury to cranial nerves may make performing these functions next to impossible. The ability to provide nutrition to a healing surgical patient is of primary concern in healing and maintenance of a patient's immune system. Early consultation may lead to early placement of percutaneous endoscopic gastrostomy feeding tubes, central catheters, and evaluation of the digestive and respiratory tracts.

## Physical therapy

The physical therapy consultation is important in the management of not only maxillofacial injuries but also any orthopedic injuries. Maxillofacial physical therapy addresses the movement of the temporomandibular joint and should address electrical stimulation of facial musculature, which has been effected by

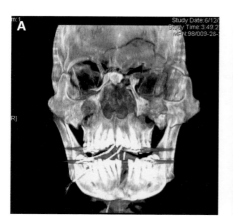
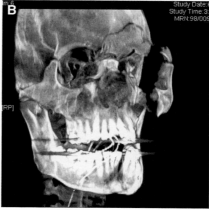

Fig. 5. (*A, B*) Examples of three-dimensional CT scans.

facial nerve injury. This stimulation prevents facial muscle atrophy and encourages facial nerve regrowth in the area of deficit.

*Pain management services*

Many patients who have returned from theater with severe injuries manage their pain with large amounts of opiate analgesics. Centrally mediated pain syndrome has been identified in a small number of patients whose pain issues have been addressed inadequately. For both of these subgroups of patients, consulting the pain management service assists in facilitating the comfort of patients and supports in the withdrawal from opiate analgesics to an appropriate level of pain medications.

## Cultures and sensitivities (infectious disease)

Casualties from OEF/OIF who have been treated in multiple health care settings, including austere combat situations, bring with them complex infectious disease issues related to multiple resistant organisms. Patients with open wounds automatically should be started on prophylactic antibiotics for 24 hours, with the cornerstone of treatment being surgical serial débridement. The decision regarding antibiotic use should be based on the area of injury and degree of wound contamination.

Should a battlefield wound become infected, treatment should be definitive, with removal of foreign bodies and necrotic and infected tissue. Empiric broad-spectrum antibiotics are initiated against likely pathogens for 7 to 10 days. Table 1 provides an overview of the various antibiotics and spectrum of coverage [7,8]. Gram stains, cultures, and sensitivities are obtained to direct antibiotic therapy. Because *Clostridium* and *Bacteroides* species are difficult to culture, antibiotic therapy should be directed to cover these organisms.

It is also important for clinicians to realize that battlefield wounds are prone to tetanus because of high levels of contamination with *C tetani*. Every effort should be made to investigate a patient's current tetanus immunization status and initiate appropriate treatment or immunization. Necrotizing soft tissue infections from clostridial myonecrosis or polymicrobial infections can be the most dangerous and lethal infections that are encountered. All layers of tissue may be involved, and the treatment involves aggressive surgical débridement combined with antibiotic therapy.

Finally, clinicians must remember that patients may present with a confusing picture because of infection of various other wounds or a progression to sepsis. Following the previously mentioned principles and maintaining vigilant monitoring during medical evacuation should allow a patient to arrive at a large tertiary care facility for more definitive treatment and reconstruction.

Table 1
Spectrum of selected antibiotic agents [16,17]

| Agent | Antibacterial spectrum |
| --- | --- |
| Penicillin G | *Streptococcus pyogenes*, penicillin-sensitive Streptococcus pneumonia, *Clostridium* sp |
| Ampicillin | Enterococcal sp, streptococcal sp, Proteus, some *Escherichia coli*, Klebsiella |
| Ampicillin/sulbactam | Enterococcal sp, streptococcal sp, Staphylococcus (not MRSA), *Escherichia coli*, Proteus, Klebsiella, *Clostridium* sp, *Bacteroides/Prevotella* sp |
| Nafcillin | Staphylococcal sp (not MRSA), streptococcal sp |
| Piperacillin/tazobactam | Enterococcal sp, streptococcal sp, Staphylococcus (not MRSA), *Escherichia coli*, *Pseudomonas* and other enterobacteriaceae, *Clostridium* sp, *Bacteroides/Prevotella* sp |
| Imipenem | Enterococcal sp, streptococcal sp, Staphylococcus(not MRSA), *Escherichia coli*, Pseudomonas and other enterobacteriaceae, *Clostridium* sp, Bacteroides/Prevotella sp |
| Cefazolin | Staphylcoccal sp(not MRSA), streptococcal sp, *Escherichia coli*, Klebsiella, Proteus |
| Ciprofloxacin | E coli, *Pseudomonas* and other enterobacteriaceae |
| Gentamycin | E coli, *Pseudomonas* and other enterobacteriaceae |
| Vancomycin | Streptococcal, enterococcal, and staphylococcal species (incl MRSA); not VRE |
| Clindamycin | *Streptococcus* sp, *Staphylococcus* sp, *Clostridium* sp, *Bacteriodes/Prevotella* sp |
| Metronidazole | *Clostridium* sp, *Bacteroides/Prevotella* sp |

*Abbreviations:* MRSA, methicillin resistant *Staphylococcus aureus*; VRE, vancomycin resistant *Enterococcus*.
*Data from* Schuster GS. The microbiology of oral and maxillofacial infections. In: Topazian RG, Goldberg MH, editors. Oral and maxillofacial infections. 3rd edition. Philadelphia: WB Saunders; 1994. p. 39–78; and Gilbert DN, Moellering Jr RC, Sande MA. The Sanford guide to antimicrobial therapy. 34th edition. Hyde Park (VT): Antimicrobial Therapy, Inc.; 2004.

Upon receipt of casualties in our facilities, culture and sensitivity for *A baumannii* automatically are initiated. A patient usually is placed in contact and airborne isolation pending results, a process that can take up to 48 hours. If this resistant organism has been cultured in patients who have returned from OIF, aggressive antibiotic therapy is initiated to include coverage with ticarcillin and an aminoglycoside. In general, comprehensive wound care management coupled with appropriate antibiotic coverage and consultation with infectious disease specialists for challenging cases can prevent life-threatening sepsis.

## Serial débridement

The role of serial débridement cannot be overstated in dealing with patients injured in combat or terrorist activities. The injury patterns seen differ in several ways from those seen in a civilian trauma setting: (1) the devastating destruction of soft and hard tissues caused by high velocity, fragmentation-type injury patterns leads to compromised tissue beyond the visibly damaged tissue; (2) the battlefield environment in which patients are injured is grossly contaminated; (3) wound care on the battlefield and while in transport is less than ideal; and (4) evacuation off the battlefield is not always expeditious, which leads to increased wound contamination. Initial wound management involves hemostasis, dressing, awaiting evacuation to an aid station, and ultimately, a higher level facility in the combat theater.

Upon presentation at a higher echelon facility, aggressive irrigation and foreign body removal and limited soft tissue débridement are completed; the wounds should be left open or packed for hemostatic

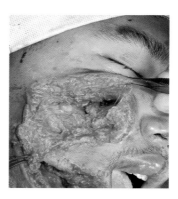

Fig. 7. Following pulsatile irrigation. (Courtesy of D. Clifford, DMD, MD; Bethesda, MD)

purposes. Tacking sutures may aid in securing gauze packing, but they should not be placed for reapproximation of wound margins. After evacuation to a higher echelon treatment facility out of theater (eg, Europe, United States), the entire wound is re-explored and débridement of grossly necrotic tissue is completed. Unless contraindicated because of concomitant injuries, aggressive irrigation with copious saline and antibiotic solution (eg, clindamycin) is performed with a pulsatile irrigation system (Pulsavac, Zimmer, Warsaw, Indiana). After the first pulsatile irrigation, superficial wet-to-dry dressing changes are performed three times per day. After 48 to 72 hours, the procedure is repeated. At that point, the surgeon is faced with the decision of when to perform the primary closure [9,10]. It has been our experience that definitive closure should not be performed if any sign of nonviable tissue is present upon exploration of the wound (Figs. 6 and 7). Delayed primary closure of the wound is generally performed after the second washout, although the threshold for continuing the débridement is low

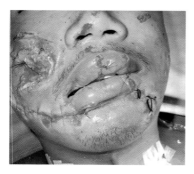

Fig. 6. Initial presentation with irrigation and débridement; tacking sutures placed. (Courtesy of D. Clifford, DMD, MD; Bethesda, MD)

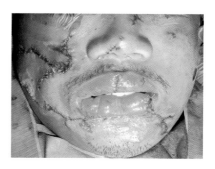

Fig. 8. Healthy appearance of tissue at time of primary closure. (Courtesy of D. Clifford, DMD, MD; Bethesda, MD)

(Fig. 8). Generally the hard tissue base is stabilized at the time of primary closure.

## Stabilization of hard tissue base to support soft tissue envelope and prevent scar contracture before primary reconstruction

Because of the high risk of infection and extensive soft tissue injury in these patients, definitive reconstruction is often deferred to a secondary phase. Our experience has demonstrated that with a lack of bony support, fibrous tissue and scar contracture compromise the eventual functional and aesthetic result of any reconstruction. In the routine trauma setting, bone grafting or alloplastic implants may be placed at the initial surgery with immediate soft tissue coverage. We have opted to use standard rigid fixation systems to span bony gaps and give support to overlying soft tissue with only limited bone grafting or other alloplast use (eg, Medpor Porex, Newnan, Georgia) as necessary to reduce scar contracture. Complete reconstruction is often deferred to a secondary phase. The placement of rigid fixation follows standard trauma protocol to provide support of the facial pillars. One of the risks of using titanium plates in this manner is that of plate exposure. Although it occurred in some patients, the associated morbidity was low, the area was excised, and primary closure was performed with minimal cosmetic defect. Another option for supporting the soft tissue is the application of an external fixator, which has proved successful in projecting the mandible and zygomaticomaxillary complexes until the primary reconstruc-

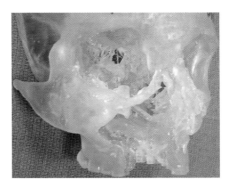

Fig. 10. Stereolithographic model demonstrates avulsive defect of midface region seen in Fig. 9. (Courtesy of D. Clifford, DMD, MD; Bethesda, MD)

tion can be undertaken. Such support also maintains a tissue plane, which provides easier dissection upon secondary reconstruction with either autogenous or alloplastic materials.

## Comprehensive review of stereolithography models and radiographs and determination of treatment goals

The ultimate treatment goal for our combat casualties with facial injuries is the restoration of function and cosmesis. Most injured patients have significant avulsive defects of facial structures. CT scans are the gold standard for imaging of facial fractures (Fig. 9). Three-dimensional reconstructed CT scans and stereolithographic models are essential adjunctive elements in preparing a treatment plan for avulsive-type defects (Fig. 10). The most important aspect of treating avulsive defects is using appropriate imaging to develop a staged reconstruction plan with the final endpoint in mind before any reconstruction begins. Items for consideration in viewing the studies and models are (1) which structures are missing, (2) which structures remain, (3) the effect of each on the reconstruction goals, (4) which structures require replacement, (5) how those structures will be replaced (nonvascularized versus vascularized tissue), (6) identifying stabilization points for replacement structures, (7) soft tissue considerations, (8) choice of grafting material, and (9) the effect of grafting plan on future implant reconstruction or dental rehabilitation. The choice of grafting or replacement material includes (1) bone (eg, cranial, iliac crest [block versus particulate], osteomyocutnaeous vascularized flaps), (2) myocutaneous

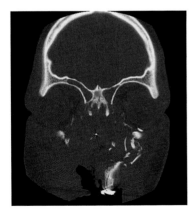

Fig. 9. CT scan demonstrates avulsive defect of midface region. (Courtesy of D. Clifford, DMD, MD; Bethesda, MD)

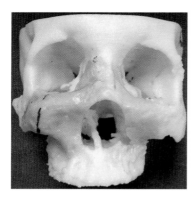

Fig. 11. Replacement of avulsed tissue with wax for template formation. (Courtesy of J. Solomon, DMD and G. Waskewicz, DDS; Bethesda, MD)

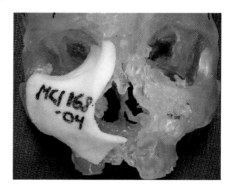

Fig. 13. Custom Medpor implant for avulsive midface defect seen in Figs. 9 and 10. (Courtesy of D. Clifford, DMD, MD; Bethesda, MD)

vascularized flaps, and (3) alloplast. Stereolitho-graphic models allow for wax replacement of avulsed structures (Fig. 11) or generation of mirror-image structures, prebending of plates (Fig. 12), fabrication of templates for contouring of bone grafts, fabrication of custom implants (Fig. 13) (Medpor Porex, Newnan, Georgia, titanium, or polymethylmethacrylate), or use of stock alloplasts (eg, Medpor) [5].

### Replacement of missing soft tissue component

If soft tissue has been avulsed or is lost over the course of serial débridement, it is absolutely critical to replace this tissue with some form of vascularized flap—either rotational flap or free flap—before the development of scar contractures or colonization with

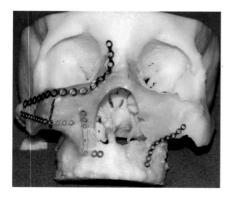

Fig. 12. Plates prebent to wax template replacing avulsed tissue. (Courtesy of J. Solomon, DMD and G. Waskewicz, DDS; Bethesda, MD)

bacteria from the oral cavity or external environment (Fig. 14). Once scar contractures develop, it is essentially impossible to recover from this and create a normal soft tissue appearance. In our experience, vascularized tissue is more resistant to secondary infection and scar contracture and gives the most ideal result. Patients who present with injuries sustained by IED blasts usually are already contaminated with multiple bacterial species and are highly susceptible to recurrent infections and secondary scarring. The use of vascularized tissue has helped minimize complications in these cases. When faced with the dilemma of using a local rotational flap versus free flap, the reconstructive surgeon should determine whether a satisfactory result can be obtained in one surgical procedure or if several revision surgeries are necessary (Fig. 15). If a single surgery is planned, rotation of a local flap may be indicated because of the similarities in tissue coloration, consistency, and appearance. If the need for future surgical intervention is necessary, consideration should be given to using the free tissue transfer initially to inhibit scar contracture and finalize treatment at the secondary and tertiary surgeries with the local flap (Fig. 16). We recommend waiting a minimum of 8 to 12 weeks after placement of a graft to allow for maturation before the next surgical procedure at that site (Fig. 17).

### Primary reconstruction and fracture management

The goal of primary reconstruction should be to obtain the best functional and cosmetic results possible, because the tissues injured by explosive projectiles may have significant scar contracture at

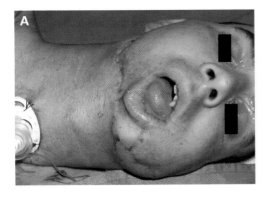
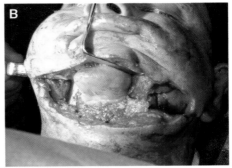

Fig. 14. (*A*) Presurgical appearance. Soft tissue closure accomplished at field hospital. (*B*) Avulsive injury with significant loss of soft tissue.

any future procedure and the opportunity to obtain a satisfactory result will be decreased. Preoperative planning is of paramount importance, with support of the soft tissue envelope being a priority for maintaining as normal a facial contour as possible.

Replacement of missing bone should be included in this treatment planning, because support of the soft tissue envelope is important. A strong recommendation is to consider exhausting native bone graft options before resorting to other choices. If the

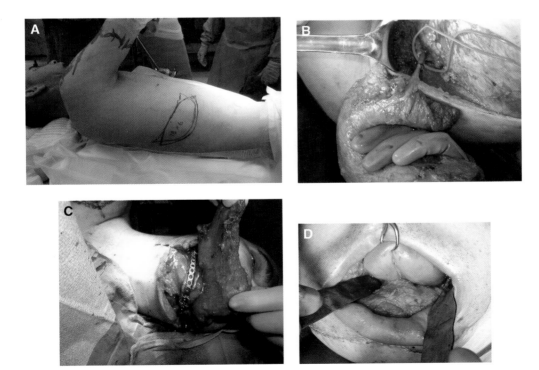

Fig. 15. (*A*) Location of latissimus dorsi free flap donor site. (*B*) Mobilization of the flap and preservation of vascular access. (*C*) Latissimus dorsi free tissue transfer to the mandibular region. The vascular supply is from the superior thyroid artery. Note presence of reconstruction bar to provide support to the free flap and assist with prevention of scar contracture. Osseous reconstruction is attempted at secondary surgery with corticocancellous bone graft. (*D*) Reconstruction of the floor of mouth with the muscular component of the latissimus dorsi flap.

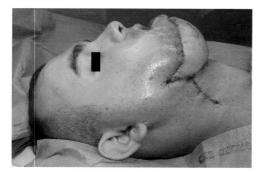

Fig. 16. Appearance of flap immediately postoperatively.

recipient site is contaminated or infected, which is not unlikely in cases of IED blasts, our experiences have shown that allogeneic bone has a high propensity for resorption and chronic foreign body reaction. Native bone, particularly bone transferred with periosteal coverage, has been less likely to show evidence of late infection and better maintains the soft tissue projection obtained. In cases of significant panfacial trauma that involves the maxilla and mandible, we recommend sequencing of treatment as previously published by Wong and Johnson (Box 2) [11].

Our clinical experience has been to secure the airway and reconstruct the mandible as a first stage in surgery. In most cases of panfacial fractures, accomplishing these procedures takes several hours at a minimum, and proceeding immediately to a lengthy reconstruction of the midface and orbital fractures may not be advised because of potential fatigue of the surgical team. Breaking after the mandibular proce-

dures also allows for dental impressions and splint fabrication to occur to a known reference point, the newly reconstructed mandible.

One of the more common errors associated with panfacial trauma reconstruction is inadequate reduction of the mandibular archform, which results in excessive facial width secondary to splaying of the mandibular angles [12]. Excessive width of the mandibular angles results in the appearance of retrognathia because of posterior positioning of the mandibular symphysis. If the mandible is plated in the wrong position, ultimately the maxilla and zygomaticomaxillary complex also are improperly positioned, which results in excessive width to the face and the appearance of midfacial deficiency. This complication can be prevented by using prebent surgical plates made from stereolithographic or cadaveric/anatomic models to ensure accurate gonial width and anterior projection of the mandibular symphysis (Fig. 18).

After proper fixation of the mandible, attention is directed to zygomaticomaxillary complex and arch projection. Our experience has been that accurate positioning of the malar prominence and zygomatic arch is best accomplished by direct visualization of the zygomaticomaxillary and zygomaticotemporal

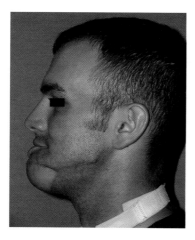

Fig. 17. Appearance of patient 4 months after free flap.

Box 2. Sequencing of treatment for panfacial trauma

  Secure definitive airway
  Obain reduction and fixation of mandibular fractures
  Obtain mandibular arch impressions for fabrication of occlusal/palatal splints as necessary using the fixed mandible as template
  Position LeFort fractures into occlusion with mandibular dentition using maxillomandibular fixation
  Obtain reproducible seating of mandibular condyles into fossa
  Repair frontal sinus fractures if present
  Reduce zygomatic complexes and reconstruct nasofrontal junction
  Reduce naso-orbital-ethmoid complex fractures and medial canthopexies
  Reduce infraorbital rims
  Reduce LeFort I level fractures
  Reduce orbital floor fractures
  Undertake nasal grafting

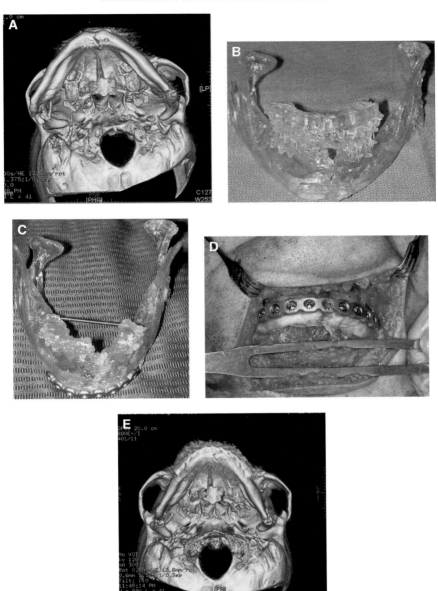

Fig. 18. (*A*) Three-dimensional CT scan shows excessive widening of the mandibular angles before definitive treatment of mandibular fractures. Anterior symphysis plate currently serves to stabilize fracture segments. Note open lingual cortical plate. (*B*) Stereolithography model of radiograph shown in (*A*). (*C*) Stereolithography model is sectioned and repositioned in accordance with accepted anatomic norms for gonial distance and ramus distance. Reconstruction bar is prebent to new dimensions to correctly position the segments intraoperatively. Condylar fracture reduction occurs during the same operation to correct vertical and anteroposterior position of the mandible before treatment of maxillary fractures. (*D*) Intraoperative view of mandibular fracture reduction and positioning of reconstruction bar. Proper positioning of mandibular angles is obtained by the surgical assistant, who places pressure in the region of the mandibular angles until fractured segments passively fit the reconstruction bar. The gonial distance was reduced 2.5 cm in this case from the presurgical dimensions. (*E*) Postoperative three-dimensional CT scan shows improved dimensions of gonial distance and mandibular contour and shape. Proper reduction of midfacial fractures can occur at this time to optimize aesthetic and functional result.

junctions by the use of the coronal flap (Fig. 19). Some surgeons may argue that the scar from the coronal flap is unsightly and an "acceptable" position of the zygomaticomaxillary complex can be obtained by other approaches. In cases of minimal or isolated fractures of the zygomaticomaxillary complex we would agree. Our bias in cases of significant midfacial destruction or gross comminution of the maxilla is that proper projection of the midface cannot occur without direct visualization, and ultimately secondary scar contracture continues to displace the segments and results in the previously "acceptable" appearance ultimately becoming unacceptable. Our technique is to use the stereolithographic model as a template for plate adaptation. If the contralateral side is unaffected, we bend surgical plates to that side of the model and place them on the affected side whenever possible to reproduce accurately a patient's preinjury skeletal contours and maximize the potential for an accurate zygomatic width and good soft tissue projection after healing.

When properly designed and positioned, the coronal flap can be aesthetically pleasing. Our technique involves placing approximately 10 cc of 2% lidocaine with 1:100,000 epinephrine along the proposed incision site. We place the local anesthesia before performing the surgical scrub and address any obvious sources of vascular bleeding with cautious application of electrocautery. After reflection of the flap, a moist surgical sponge is placed over the cut edges to prevent desiccation at the incision edge and assist with control of bleeding. Blood loss in all cases has been minimal. This technique has been used in more than 20 cases by one of the authors and eliminates the need for scalp clips, which prevents

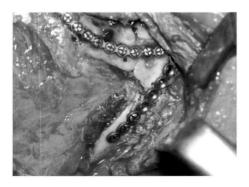

Fig. 19. Accurate reproduction of zygomaticomaxillary complex and zygomatic arch accomplished by prebending surgical plates on contralateral side of stereolithography model to reproduce preinjury facial projection and use of coronal flap for access.

possible formation of traumatic alopecia that can occur during prolonged reconstruction cases.

## Aggressive physical and occupational therapy

Oral and maxillofacial disability can result from scar contracture, soft or hard tissue fibrosis, and muscle atrophy caused by prolonged maxillomandibular fixation. Injured soldiers returning from OIF/OEF often present with some degree of maxillofacial disability. The injuries sustained typically involve soft tissue and hard tissue loss and comminution of the facial bony structure.

Soft tissue fibrosis and scar contracture are typically seen weeks to months after injury repair [13,14]. Initial management after adequate healing involves mandibular opening exercises with lateral excursive movements. The patients also perform manual massage of the injured area in an effort to soften fibrosis and contracture bands. The goal of this modality is to reduce the soft tissue tension and allow a full range of mandibular movement [15]. If this conservative therapy is not successful, a more aggressive regimen is followed to include a commercially available mandibular functional device. Our institutions use the Therabite device (Atos Medical AB, Hörby, Sweden) for cases that require further therapy. The protocol for this device is seven mandibular stretches held at maximum opening for 7 seconds. This routine is repeated seven times daily until a patient achieves a maximum incisal opening larger than 35 mm or improvement is no longer achieved. Another modality of therapy for soft tissue fibrosis involves injection of steroids into the fibrotic area. This approach promotes the reconfiguration of collagen fibrils and softening of the scar, which releases the tension of the soft tissue. Mandibular function is reassessed after 4 to 6 months of healing and therapy. For areas with high tension that have not responded to prior interventions, scar revision is considered with excision of fibrotic tissue and soft tissue release using rotational flaps or undermining procedures. Emphasis is placed on tension-free closure to allow optimal healing with minimal scarring.

Hard tissue fibrosis is seen in patients who sustain maxillofacial injuries caused by the degree of bone destruction and secondary blast effects. Patients with severe comminution of the mandible or maxilla typically undergo maxillomandibular fixation for 6 weeks. After the release of fixation, patients typically demonstrate a maximum incisal opening smaller than

15 mm [13,14]. Patients are instructed on active mandibular range-of-motion exercises and manual techniques to aid in opening. These exercises are performed with minimal pressure so as not to affect the healing fracture. For patients who do not respond to mandibular opening or manual manipulation, the Therabite device is introduced to their routine and the standard protocol is used. For patients with mandibular disability secondary to temporalis fibrosis who do not respond to conservative therapy, coronoidectomies may be considered. The goal of this intervention is to release the temporalis muscle attachment to the mandible and allow normal mandibular function.

Because of the destructive nature of the injuries sustained by soldiers in support of OIF/OEF, many casualties with oral and maxillofacial injuries present with mandibular disability secondary to either soft tissue or hard tissue fibrosis. The management approach to these patients—after all injuries are healed—follows a conservative algorithm with escalation as needed to achieve normal mandibular function. For this approach to be successful, patient compliance is necessary with diligence in following instructions as prescribed.

## Secondary reconstruction

The primary purposes of secondary reconstructive procedures should be to increase functional activity of the maxillofacial complex, correct obvious errors or bony relapses from the primary surgical intervention, and improve the cosmetic appearance of a patient. As with any trauma patient, a surgeon should begin to formulate the long-term reconstruction plans before any surgical treatment to avoid performing procedures that may limit definitive reconstruction. As many authors have expressed and we have emphasized repeatedly in this article, the success of long-term reconstruction depends greatly on initial wound management and the prevention of scar contracture. The ideal end result of the reconstructive process is to restore a patient to a functional dentition with optimal cosmesis. With avulsion of tissue associated with high-energy injury patterns, we have found that definitive reconstruction of the jaws is limited by the hard and soft tissue defect and the associated scarring, which often requires numerous secondary procedures. Common procedures performed during this phase from the maxillofacial surgery perspective include placement of ocular, auricular, or dental implants for prosthetic replacement or preprosthetic surgery wholly for dental

indications, such as vestibuloplasty, ridge augmentation, alveolar distraction, or orthognathic surgery to correct maxillary-mandibular arch discrepancies.

In dealing with soft tissue injuries as seen in terrorist attacks or warfare, a surgeon must show some creativity while maintaining basic surgical principles. Replacement of soft tissue can be as simple as skin grafting or local flap advancement, or it can be as advanced as tissue expansion or free flaps. Microstomia secondary to tissue loss or scarring may be addressed initially to give better access for intraoral procedures, which may be a necessity for dental impressions to be taken. Intraoral fibrous scar bands can be excised and grafts placed. In areas that have suffered from avulsive injuries, local recruitment of tissues should be the first option, with regional or free flaps used when the local tissues are inadequate. Free gingival grafts or connective tissue grafts are performed to restore an adequate amount of attached gingiva. After the primary bone grafting is complete, a prosthodontic consultation should be obtained for definitive treatment planning. A maxillofacial prosthodontist should be involved early in the treatment of large avulsive injuries, notably when an obturator for maxillary defects is proposed.

## Posttraumatic scarring and cosmetic management

Complex maxillofacial penetrating trauma related to blast and ballistic injuries frequently results in aggressive, disfiguring scars. The combination of a high degree of wound contamination, wound avulsion, and loss of tissue vitality contributes to significant cicatrix formation and facial disfigurement. Our experiences managing these complex wounds sustained by servicemen and servicewomen in support of OIF and OEF have served as a basis for the following discussion according to the lessons learned by our surgeons.

The key to a successful cosmetic outcome after these devastating injuries is based on intervening procedures designed to prevent cicatrix formation rather than strictly addressing wound scarring as a secondary procedure. Initial management of these injuries must include early, extensive wound débridement of contamination through serial "wash outs" with copious antibiotic-containing irrigation solutions and obtaining wound cultures along the way to identify infective organisms and their appropriate sensitivities. Assessment of the degree of missing tissue present after these blast injuries is imperative. Patients who present with tissue loss or avulsion that is left to heal secondarily will develop severe disfiguring scar formation. Early identification of tissue loss followed by procedures to bring vascularized tissue through local rotation flaps or distant free flaps is essential to minimize scarring and maximize form and function. Early reduction and fixation of underlying bony fractures and replacement of missing osseous structures with bone grafts or alloplastic augmentation also are essential for a favorable return of form and function and minimization of cicatrix formation. Early intervention regarding reconstruction of the underling bony defects and overlying cutaneous defects should b accomplished within 10 to 14 days of injury to avoid extensive wound contracture and aggressive scarring. This is certainly a reasonable time period to initiate these surgical procedures once appropriate consultations have been accomplished and wound infection has been ruled out or appropriately treated. If this protocol is followed, the resultant scar formation should be minimized and amenable to the following treatment options to accomplish a cosmetically acceptable outcome.

Scarring associated with ballistic and blast injuries usually presents with tattooing of the penetrated tissues secondary to impregnation of the skin by metallic fragments. In addition to the tattoo effect, there is usually hypertophic cicatrix formation. Early program dermabrasion of these scars 4 to 6 weeks after soft tissue closure or scar excision/revision has proved to be beneficial to leveling the skin and improving cosmesis. Injecting subcutaneous kenalog to reduce hypertrophic scarring is also beneficial as long as long as low doses are used so as not to cause significant dermal atrophy or liponecrosis. Topical application of silastic gel or sheets through a relatively unknown mechanism also improves wound levels and cosmesis. Topical application of imiquimod 5% cream also has been reported to reduce hypertrophic scar formation by activating cellular cytokines and alpha interferon. This agent is helpful if initiated by the second week after the wound repair [16].

Tattooing of the skin with gray-blue pigmentation after penetrating metallic injury can be reduced significantly or eliminated with treatments using the pulsed-dye laser. The pulsed dye laser (595 nm, yellow light laser) provides collagen rebuilding and reorganization while normalizing neovascularization. These treatments can be repeated on a monthly basis for eight to ten applications. The tattooing is secondary to implanted metallic fragments that consist of copper, zinc, graphite, and other metals. The metallic fragments can be disrupted through "photo acoustic shattering" of the pigmented particles using a "Q-switched" laser. Two other lasers have been effective in our experience in reducing tattooing: the Nd Yag (1064 nm) infrared laser and the red Alexandrite laser (755 nm). We are convinced that persistence of these foreign particles within the soft tissues provides the impetus and etiology for significant hypertophic scar formation. Prompt scar excision and revision coupled with laser-assisted phagocytosis and elimination of metallic particles provide the greatest likelihood of a favorable cosmetic soft tissue wound result [17].

Facial scarring secondary to ballistic and blast-related injuries is a significant cosmetic concern. The outcome can be made more predictable and cosmetically pleasing if certain treatment protocols and modalities are used. Essential considerations must include early fixation and reconstitution of the facial skeleton, followed by passive soft tissue wound closure through use of local rotational flaps or distant free flaps. In our experience, early scar excision and revision along with early program dermabrasion and use of laser technology to remove tattooing of soft tissue seem to provide the most favorable cosmetic outcome for these devastating facial injuries. Measures used to prevent or eliminate wound contamination and contraction provide the foundation for the most favorable cosmetic outcome. Preventive measures always outweigh the benefits of secondary management of posttraumatic scarring.

## Summary

The management of complex maxillofacial injuries sustained in modern warfare or terrorist attack has presented military surgeons with a new form of injury pattern previously not discussed in the medical literature. The unique wounding characteristics of the IED, the portability of the weapon platform, and the relative low cost of development make it an ideal weapon for potential terrorist attacks. If potential future terrorist attacks in the United States follow the same pattern as the incidents currently unfolding in the Middle East, civilian practitioners will be required to manage these wounds early for primary surgical intervention and late for secondary and tertiary reconstructive efforts.

The use of stereolithographic models in presurgical planning of complex maxillofacial injuries is critical and should be considered the standard of care. These models can be manufactured during the initial 48- to 72-hour period of serial débridement and surgical washouts. They are invaluable in visualizing the bony architecture of the skeletal framework. Our experiences with patients injured by IED blasts indicate that they are highly likely to become infected by some type of organism, the only variable being when the infection will develop over the course of treatment. Scar contracture that occurs either secondary to infection or as a consequence of improper positioning of the bony substructure of the face is almost impossible to recover from if inadequate projection of the soft tissue envelope is not maintained. The treating surgeon should not fall victim to the mistake of rushing these patients to the operating room for definitive treatment before gathering the appropriate preoperative data. Projection and support of the soft tissue envelope is critical to the success of any surgical treatment initially performed. We also have used this treatment protocol on civilian panfacial trauma casualties, such as victims of automobile accidents or isolated gunshot wounds, and have found it to be successful. Whereas our wish is that the information presented in this article never will be used in the United States for the treatment of patients injured in another terrorist attack, the lessons learned in the management of modern ballistic injuries and wounds sustained in warfare should be shared with the civilian community so that if that day ever comes, we shall all be prepared.

## Acknowledgments

The authors would like to acknowledge the chief residents of the National Capitol Consortium Oral and Maxillofacial Surgery Training Program, Michael J. Doherty, DDS, and Charles G. Stone, Jr, DDS, for their assistance with the research and preparation of this article.

## References

[1] Sakula A. Sir Harold Gillies, FRCS (1882–1960). J Med Biogr 2004;12(2):65.

[2] Triana Jr RJ. Sir Harold Gillies. Arch Facial Plast Surg 1999;1(2):142–3.

[3] Shaolin Wahnam Institute. Quotes from famous warriors. Available at: http://wongkiewkit.com/forum/showthread.php?t=642. Accessed April 18, 2005.

[4] Robertson BC, Manson PN. High-energy ballistic and avulsive injuries: a management protocol for the next millennium. Surg Clin North Am 1999;79(6): 1489–502.

[5] Powers DB, Edgin WA, Tabatchnick L. Stereolithography: a historical review and indications for use in the management of trauma. J Craniomaxillofac Trauma 1998;4(3):16–23.

[6] Scott PT, Peterson K, Fishbain J, et al. Acinetobacter baumannii infections among patients at military medical facilities treating injured US service members, 2002–2004. MMWR Morb Mortal Wkly Rep 2004; 53(45):1063–6.

[7] Schuster GS. The microbiology of oral and maxillofacial infections. In: Topazian RG, Goldberg MH, editors. Oral and maxillofacial infections. 3rd edition. Philadelphia: WB Saunders; 1994. p. 39–78.

[8] Gilbert DN, Moellering Jr RC, Sande MA. The Sanford guide to antimicrobial therapy. 34th edition. Hyde Park (VT): Antimicrobial Therapy, Inc.; 2004.

[9] Eppley BL, Bhuller A. Principles of facial soft tissue repair. In: Booth PW, Eppley B, Schmelzheisen R, editors. Maxillofacial trauma and esthetic facial reconstruction. Edinburgh: Churchill-Livingstone; 2003. p. 107–20.

[10] Clark N, Birely B, Manson PN, et al. High-energy ballistic and avulsive facial injuries: classification, patterns, and an algorithm for primary reconstruction. Plast Reconstr Surg 1996;98(4):583–601.

[11] Wong MEK, Johnson JV. Management of midface injuries. In: Fonseca RJ, editor. Oral and maxillofacial surgery. 1st edition. Philadelphia: WB Saunders; 2000. p. 245–99.

[12] Ellis E, Tharanon W. Facial width problems associated with rigid fixation of mandibular fractures: case reports. J Oral Maxillofac Surg 1992;50(1):87–94.

[13] Dolwick MF, Armstrong JW. Complications in temporomandibular joint surgery. In: Kaban LB, Pogrel MA, Perrott DH, editors. Complications in oral and maxillofacial surgery. Philadelphia: WB Saunders; 1997. p. 98–9.

[14] Keith DA. The long-term unfavorable result in temporomandibular joint surgery. In: Kaban LB, Pogrel MA, Perrott DH, editors. Complications in oral and maxillofacial surgery. Philadelphia: WB Saunders; 1997. p. 301–2.

[15] Van Sickles JE, Parks Jr WJ. Temporomandibular joint region injuries. In: Fonseca RJ, editor. Oral and maxillofacial surgery. 1st edition. Philadelphia: WB Saunders; 2000. p. 146–7.

[16] Berman B. Pilot study of the effect of postoperative imiquimod 5% cream on the recurrence rate of excised keloids. J Am Acad Dermatol 2002;47:S209–11.

[17] Maggio K. Clinical experience, laser and cutaneous surgery center. Washington, DC: Walter Reed Army Medical Center; 2004.

ELSEVIER
SAUNDERS

Oral Maxillofacial Surg Clin N Am 17 (2005) 357–363

ORAL AND
MAXILLOFACIAL
SURGERY CLINICS
of North America

# Index

*Note:* Page numbers of article titles are in **boldface** type.

## A

Airway management, in battlefield injuries, 331–332, 336
  in facial burns, 269–270
  in maxillofacial injuries, due to improvised explosive devices, 283

Alpha viruses, in biologic warfare. *See* Bioterrorism.

Amifostine, for radiation injuries, due to terrorist attacks, 295

Angiogenesis, in wound healing, 243

Anthrax, in bioterrorism. *See* Bioterrorism.

Anthrax meningitis, in bioterrorism, 308

Antibiotics, for plague, 312–313
  for Q fever, 320
  for tularemia, 317

Arenavirus. *See* Bioterrorism, viral hemorrhagic fevers in.

Argentine hemorrhagic fever. *See* Bioterrorism, viral hemorrhagic fevers in.

Asphyxiation, in inhalation burns, 268–269

Avulsive gunshot wounds, healing of, 247

## B

*Bacillus anthracis. See* Bioterrorism, anthrax in.

Ballistic injuries, **251–259**
  at close range versus distance, 257–258
  caliber of projectile in, 251–252
  exit versus entrance wounds in, 258
  full metal jacketed bullets in, 254–255
  high-velocity projectiles in, 255–256
    versus low-velocity projectiles, 252–254
    yaw in, 256–257
  magnum cartridges in, 252
  sterility of projectiles in, 258

Bicarbonate, for radiation injuries, due to terrorist attacks, 295

Biologic warfare. *See* Bioterrorism.

Bioterrorism, **299–330**
  alpha viruses in, 324
    clinical features of, 324
    diagnosis of, 324
    infection control and prevention in, 324
    management of, 324
    virology of, 324
  and oral and maxillofacial surgeon, 324–325
  anthrax in, 306–311
    anthrax meningitis, 308
    cutaneous, 307, 308, 309
    diagnosis of, 308–309
    differential diagnosis of, 308–309
    epidemiology of, 306–307
    gastrointestinal, 307–308
    historical aspects of, 300, 306
    infection control and prevention in, 309–311
    inhalational, 308, 309–311
    management of, 309
    microbiology of, 307–308
  biologic weapons proliferation in, 300–301
  botulinum toxin in, 313–315
    diagnosis of, 315
    differential diagnosis of, 315
    epidemiology of, 313–314
    historical aspects of, 313
    infection control and prevention in, 315
    management of, 315
    microbiology of, 314
    pathogenesis and clinical features of, 314
  brucellosis in, 320–321
    diagnosis of, 321
    epidemiology of, 321
    historical aspects of, 320
    management of, 321
    microbiology of, 321
    pathogenesis and clinical features of, 321
  future directions in, 325–326
  future threats of, assessment of, 326
  historical aspects of, 299–300

# Changing Your Address?

Make sure your subscription changes too! When you notify us of your new address, you can help make our job easier by including an exact copy of your Clinics label number with your old address (see illustration below.) This number identifies you to our computer system and will speed the processing of your address change. Please be sure this label number accompanies your old address and your corrected address—you can send an old Clinics label with your number on it or just copy it exactly and send it to the address listed below.

We appreciate your help in our attempt to give you continuous coverage. Thank you.

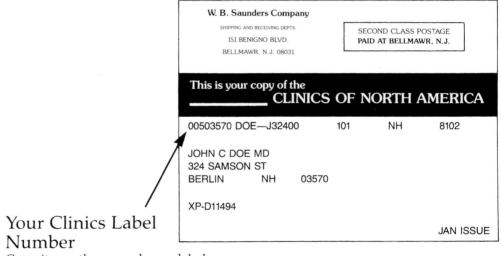

## Your Clinics Label Number
Copy it exactly or send your label along with your address to:
**W.B. Saunders Company, Customer Service**
Orlando, FL 32887-4800
Call Toll Free 1-800-654-2452

Please allow four to six weeks for delivery of new subscriptions and for processing address changes.